1. A pain in your lower right or left side can be a sign of ovulation. True or false?

2. Is abdominal pain a symptom of cancer?

3. When is severe abdominal pain a sign of a life-threatening problem?

4. Is persistent indigestion cause for worry?

5. What is the optimal amount of fiber to eat a day?

6. What pain is the most frequent cause of a doctor visit?

7. Which type of laxative is safest?

ISN'T IT IMPORTANT THAT YOU HAVE THE FACTS? YOUR LIFE AND YOUR HEALTH MAY DEPEND ON THEM.

Answers:

1. *True.*

2. *Yes, but less commonly than other symptoms.*

3. *In ectopic pregnancy.*

4. *Yes, it can indicate a serious underlying disease such as ulcers or cancer.*

5. *20 grams, or the amount in 8 to 12 servings of fresh fruit, vegetables, and whole grains.*

6. *Stomachache.*

7. *Bulk laxatives.*

Books by the American Medical Women's Association

THE WOMEN'S COMPLETE HEALTHBOOK
THE AMWA GUIDE TO NUTRITION
AND WELLNESS
THE AMWA GUIDE TO PREGNANCY AND
CHILDBIRTH
THE AMWA GUIDE TO FERTILITY AND
REPRODUCTIVE HEALTH
THE AMWA GUIDE TO EMOTIONAL HEALTH
THE AMWA GUIDE TO SEXUALITY
THE AMWA GUIDE TO CANCER AND
PAIN MANAGEMENT
THE AMWA GUIDE TO AGING AND WELLNESS
THE AMWA GUIDE TO EARS,
NOSE, AND THROAT
THE AMWA GUIDE TO CARDIOVASCULAR HEALTH
THE AMWA GUIDE TO INTERNAL DISORDERS

The American Medical Women's Association

Guide to Internal Disorders

Medical Co-editors
**Roselyn Payne Epps, M.D., M.P.H.,
M.A., F.A.A.P.
Susan Cobb Stewart, M.D., F.A.C.P.**

A Dell Book

Published by
Dell Publishing
a division of
Bantam Doubleday Dell Publishing Group, Inc.
1540 Broadway
New York, New York 10036

This material was originally published along with other material in THE WOMEN'S COMPLETE HEALTHBOOK published by Delacorte Press.

Illustrations by Wendy Frost

ISBN: 0-440-22317-2

Reprinted by arrangement with Delacorte Press

Printed in the United States of America

Published simultaneously in Canada

January 1997

10 9 8 7 6 5 4 3 2 1

OPM

The AMWA Guide to Internal Disorders

Roselyn Payne Epps, M.D., M.P.H., M.A.,
and Susan Cobb Stewart, M.D.

Whether monitoring personal health care or taking care of family members, women need a definitive resource for accurate, dependable, and up-to-date information. Abdominal discomfort—often mistaken for a "stomachache"—is one of the most common complaints heard by doctors and caregivers. The abdominal cavity contains three major organ system: the digestive, urinary, and reproductive systems. *The AMWA Guide to Internal Disorders* presents precise descriptions of these systems and information about the disorders that can occur within them, as researched by the American Medical Women's Association (AMWA), the most historic and prestigious association of women physicians in the United States.

AMWA believes that women must avoid a disease-oriented approach to health and focus on maintaining optimal health on a daily and long-term basis. The more one knows about one's body and its functions, the better equipped one will be to safeguard good health through strategies such as eating properly and exercising regularly. The content of *The AMWA Guide to Internal Disorders* is organized into three major sections, each of which stresses the importance of preventive medicine and encourages total body awareness to avoid future health problems relating to the digestive, urinary, and reproductive systems.

Part I, The Reproductive System, describes in detail the female reproductive organs and their intricate functions. Understanding these systems as they develop through maturity is crucial for those who need to identify potential disorders, contemplate pregnancy, or work with one's physician to treat pain and disorders. The authors recommend preventive strategies, such as performing regular self-examinations and recognizing atypical symptoms, for maintaining good reproductive health. They advise patients on how to treat and cope with illnesses of the system.

Part II, The Kidneys and the Urinary System, provides a thorough description of this set of organs, which is fundamental to the body's ability to remove waste products and toxins from the bloodstream. Malfunctions in the kidneys, bladder, or urethra can manifest themselves in a wide variety of conditions such as bloody urine, painful infections, stones and polyps, or even acute renal failure. Preventive measures, such as keeping the blood pressure under control with a low-sodium diet, can help lower the likelihood of bladder and kidney complications. This section covers the most common symptoms, diagnoses, and treatments of the urinary system.

Part III, The Digestive System, educates the reader about the complex structures and functions of the esophagus, stomach, small and large intestines, liver, gallbladder, and pancreas. These organs digest food and absorb nutrients, which are then used to fuel all bodily functions. Problems such as diarrhea and heartburn can often be treated by eating more fiber or avoiding irritating foods; however, other problems such as cirrhosis and hepatitis require serious medical attention and aggressive treatment.

The AMWA Guide to Internal Disorders provides authoritative information that all women need to maintain good health. It illuminates the health concerns unique to women of the 1990s and offers sound medical advice. Supported by the expertise and experience of the American Medical Women's Association, *The AMWA Guide to Internal Disorders* is a progressive and comprehensive approach to health maintenance and wellness for women of all ages.

CONTENTS

PART I:
THE REPRODUCTIVE SYSTEM
Katherine A. O'Hanlan, M.D., F.A.C.O.G., F.A.C.S, and Jean L. Fourcroy, M.D., Ph.D.

Structure and Function   2
Keeping the System Healthy   10
Symptoms   18
Conditions and Disorders   19
Procedures for Women   60

PART II:
THE KIDNEYS AND THE URINARY SYSTEM
Tamara G. Bavendam, M.D., F.A.C.S, and Sandra P. Levison, M.D., F.A.C.P.

How the Urinary System Works   70
Keeping the Urinary System Healthy   72
Common Urinary Problems   75
Common Conditions Affecting the Urinary Tract   79
Infections   79
Irritations and Inflammations   82
Stones   85
Urinary Incontinence   89
Kidney Failure (Renal Failure)   95
Nephrotic Syndrome   100
Transplantation—The Gift of Life   103
Inherited Kidney Disease   105
Tumors of the Urinary System   108
Systemic Disorders   109
Pregnancy and the Urinary Tract   113
Diagnostic Techniques for Urinary Problems   118
Where to Get More Information   123

PART III:
THE DIGESTIVE SYSTEM
Susan Cobb Stewart, M.D., F.A.C.P.

Structure and Function   126
Common Digestive Symptoms   130
How to Prevent Digestive Problems   136
Disorders of the Esophagus   142
Disorders of the Stomach   156
Disorders of the Intestines   163
Liver Disorders   188
Gallbladder and Bile Duct Disorders   199
Disorders of the Pancreas   203

Editors and Contributors   207

Index   209

PART I
The Reproductive System

Katherine A. O'Hanlan, M.D.,
F.A.C.O.G., F.A.C.S.,
and Jean L. Fourcroy, M.D., Ph.D.

The organs that form the reproductive system allow humans to reproduce. Men and women have different reproductive systems that work in unison to create new life. If something goes awry with the components of the female or male reproductive system, it can affect not only the ability to have children but may also cause serious disorders warranting early detection and treatment.

STRUCTURE AND FUNCTION

The reproductive and genital organs of a fetus form during the fourth week of pregnancy. At that time, nerve, blood vessel, and tissue bundles form in patterns that distinguish males from females when they are fully developed. Development of these organs in the fetus ends during the first trimester. (See Fig. 1.1)

Many of the anatomic structures in one sex correspond to those in the other. For instance, the female clitoris and the male penis are derived from the same structures, contain the same number of nerves, and are the site of intense sensitivity during sexual activity.

A child is born with male or female reproductive organs, but these organs remain undeveloped until puberty. Then a spurt of hormones causes rapid growth and development of reproductive organs, changing body structure and function and making a person capable of reproduction.

Females usually mature sexually between the ages of 10 and 14, when the ovaries begin producing the hormone estrogen. This causes the hips to widen, breasts to develop, and body hair to grow. It also triggers menstruation, the monthly cycle of bleeding that is a key part of a woman's fertility. Women continue to produce estrogen and menstruate until about age 50. The amount of estrogen produced by her ovaries slowly decreases until a woman reaches menopause, when her periods stop and she is no longer able to become pregnant naturally.

Males develop sexually a little later than females. At puberty, the hormone testosterone causes an increase in height, muscle development, and the growth of the sex organs, which then produce sperm. Boys may have nocturnal emissions of semen, or wet dreams, at puberty. Around age 50, the production of testosterone in men may decrease. Although lowered levels of testosterone do not seem to affect the ability to have an erection, it may result in a decrease in sexual desire.

The Female Reproductive System

A woman's external genital area is called the vulva. It is made up of the labia minora—the inner lips enclosing the opening to the vagina—and the labia majora—the outer, hair-bearing lips surrounding the opening of the vagina and the urethra, the opening to the bladder. The clitoris is a small bud-shaped organ, located just above the urethra. It is the most sensitive area of the external female genitals. Bartholin's glands are located on either side of the vaginal opening.

The vagina is a muscular tube leading from the external genital organs to the uterus. The opening of the uterus, the cervix, projects into the upper end of the vagina. (See Fig. 1.2) It varies in shape and size depending on whether a woman has had children. The cervix can be felt by inserting a finger into the vagina. It cannot be penetrated by a penis, a tampon, or a finger.

The uterus is a hollow, muscular organ, about the size of a pear, in which the fetus grows during pregnancy. (See Fig. 1.3) The lining of the uterus, the endometrium, changes in thickness depending on a woman's men-

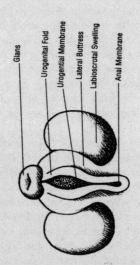

Glans

Urogenital Fold

Urogenital Membrane

Lateral Buttress

Labioscrotal Swelling

Anal Membrane

Figure 1.1 Fetal Genitalia

The fetus's external genitalia develop during early pregnancy. Both male and female genitalia arise from the same structure (top), which has begun to form by about 4-7 weeks of gestation. The *glans* gives rise to either the male glans of the penis (bottom left) or the female clitoris (bottom right). The *urogenital membrane* will eventually develop into the urethra, and the *labioscrotal swelling* will form either the male scrotum or the female labia.

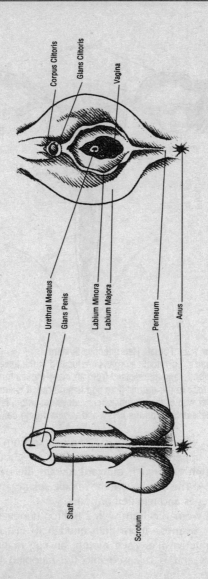

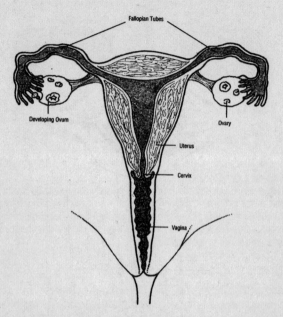

Figure 1.2   Female Reproductive System
A woman's reproductive organs are located in the lower abdomen.
Each month, an egg released from an *ovary* moves through a *fallopian tube* to the *uterus*. If an egg is fertilized, it is embedded in
the inner wall of the uterus, where it develops into a fetus. The
fetus passes through the *cervix* and *vagina* during delivery.

strual cycle. The fallopian tubes extend from either side
of the upper end of the uterus. They are about 4 inches
in length and reach outward toward the ovaries. (See
Fig. 1.4) The ovaries are the female sex organs that produce eggs and female hormones.

A woman is born with 2 million undeveloped eggs
in her ovaries—more than enough to last during her
reproductive life. Each month, an egg matures in the
ovaries and is released into the fallopian tubes. This

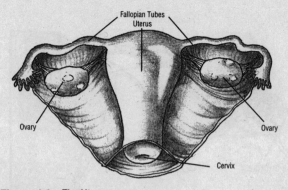

Figure 1.3 The Uterus
The uterus (seen here from the back) is a hollow, muscular organ that varies in size and shape. In women who have not had children, it usually measures about two and a half to a little over three inches long. In women who have had children, it ranges from about three and a half to four inches long.

process is called ovulation. If a man and a woman have sex at that time and the man's sperm unites with the woman's egg, fertilization occurs. The fertilized egg then moves into the woman's uterus where it becomes attached to the endometrium and begins to grow into a fetus. (See Fig. 1.5) If the egg is not fertilized, it dissolves in her body. The endometrium, which thickens before ovulation to prepare for the fertilized egg, begins to break down and menstruation, or bleeding, occurs. The hormones estrogen and progesterone, produced in the ovaries, regulate the menstrual cycle (see "Hormones of the Reproductive System").

Estrogen is secreted by the ovaries throughout a woman's reproductive years, affecting all the cells of the body. Special estrogen receptors are located in the breasts, the lining of the uterus, the cervix, and the upper vagina. Cells with estrogen receptors grow when estrogen is in the blood, whether it is secreted from the ovaries

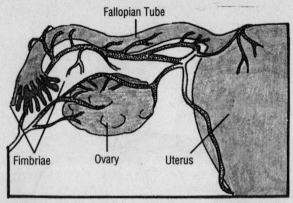

Figure 1.4 The Fallopian Tubes
The fallopian tubes extend outward from either side of the uterus. At the end of each tube, fingerlike projections called *fimbriae* are situated close to the surface of the ovary. During ovulation, the egg released by one of the ovaries enters the tube through the fimbriae.

or taken in pill form. The lining of the uterus has the greatest number of receptors, and it thickens on a monthly basis. Each month, when estrogen levels decline, the lining is broken down and results in a menstrual period.

Progesterone is a hormone secreted by the ovaries after ovulation. It causes the uterine lining cells to stop growing and to simply prepare to nourish an egg should it be fertilized and become implanted in the uterus. At menopause, when ovulation ceases, no more progesterone can be made by the ovaries.

The menstrual cycle is an average of 28 days, although some women have longer or shorter cycles. Ovulation occurs at around day 14 of the cycle (counting from the first day of the previous menstrual period), and it is at this time that a woman can become pregnant. Once released, the egg remains fertile for up to 48 hours. (See Figure 1.6)

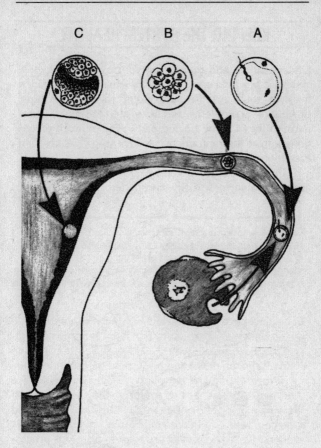

Figure 1.5 Fertilization
The process of fertilization begins with the release of an egg from one of the ovaries. Normally, penetration of an egg by a sperm occurs in the far end of a fallopian tube (A) anywhere from 12 to 24 hours after ovulation. By the time the fertilized egg has reached the near end of the tube (B), it has already begun to divide. Implantation in the wall of the uterus (C) usually occurs 3-4 days after ovulation.

KEEPING THE SYSTEM HEALTHY

Understanding and monitoring your own reproductive system is key to keeping it healthy. Health maintenance involves routine self-examinations, regular checkups, prevention of problems, and being alert to signs of problems so they can be treated early. A number of practitioners treat the reproductive system (see "Health Care Practitioners").

The reproductive systems of both women and men are vulnerable to sexually transmitted diseases (STDs),

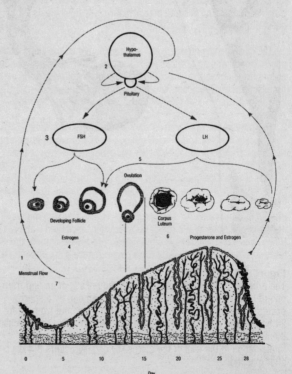

such as syphilis, gonorrhea, herpes, chlamydia, human papillomavirus (HPV), and AIDS. To protect against STDs, you should limit your sexual partners and always use a condom during sexual intercourse. A woman having sex with another woman should be careful not to have contact with her partner's genital fluids or with any open sores on her partner's body. (The use of a dental dam or cellophane wrap has been advocated but has not

Figure 1.6 The Menstrual Cycle
During the menstrual cycle, an egg is produced, released into a fallopian tube, and eventually, the uterine lining is shed if fertilization does not occur. The average menstrual cycle typically lasts 28 days, but it may vary from 23 to 35 days.

1. The cycle begins on day 1 of menstruation, when the lining of the uterus (the *endometrium*) is shed as menstrual blood. Menstruation occurs in response to a decline in the hormones estrogen and progesterone, which occurs when an egg is not fertilized.
2. The decrease in estrogen and progesterone causes the *hypothalamus* to send a message to the *pituitary*.
3. The pituitary in turn releases *follicle-stimulating hormone* (FSH). Follicles are the structures inside the ovaries that produce eggs for fertilization. Each month, one follicle will produce the egg for that cycle.
4. FSH continues to be produced during days 1-13 of the menstrual cycle. Under its influence, the developing follicle begins to produce estrogen. This hormone stimulates the endometrium to grow and thicken in preparation for a fertilized egg. At this time, the mucus normally produced by the cervix becomes thin, clear, and watery.
5. As the developing follicle continues to produce estrogen, the hormone triggers the pituitary to release *luteinizing hormone* (LH). LH stimulates the follicle to release an egg into a fallopian tube. This event, called *ovulation*, typically occurs on day 14 of the cycle.
6. After releasing the egg, the follicle begins to change into a structure known as the *corpus luteum*. This structure then begins to produce the hormone progesterone, which causes the lining of the uterus to continue to thicken in preparation for a fertilized egg.
7. If the egg is not fertilized, a sharp drop occurs in the production of estrogen and progesterone. This triggers the shedding of the endometrium, which marks the start of another menstrual cycle.

HORMONES OF THE REPRODUCTIVE SYSTEM

The reproductive systems of both women and men are regulated by hormones produced by glands that are part of the endocrine system. At the onset of puberty, the hypothalamus gland sends a signal to the pituitary gland to secrete hormones that cause the development of sexual organs.

The hypothalamus cells in the brain secrete peptides to signal the pituitary. This area regulates eating, drinking, sleeping, waking, body temperature, chemical balances, heart rate, hormones, sex, and emotions.

The pituitary, a small, gray, rounded gland attached to the base of the brain, is an endocrine gland secreting a number of hormones. The pituitary is often referred to as the master gland of the body.

Gonads (sex glands) are the testes in the male and the ovaries in the female. These glands produce the male and female hormones that regulate reproduction:

- Estrogen is the female hormone produced by the ovaries that is responsible for ovulation.

- Progesterone is a female hormone produced by the ovaries after ovulation. It triggers the menstrual period. It prepares the uterine lining for the fertilized egg.

- Testosterone is the gonadal steroid secreted by the male. After puberty, the normal male secretes testosterone daily. It is responsible for the growth of the prostate and the penis during puberty.

been shown to be as clearly of value as the condom is for heterosexuals.) In men, certain STDs can appear as an inflammation of the urethra or a discharge, but also can occur without symptoms. In women, there can be no symptoms. Both women and men should be alert to the early signs of STDs, get treatment immediately, and avoid spreading the disease to others (see "Sexually Transmitted Diseases").

Every woman's genitals are shaped individually, with different sizes for inner lips, outer lips, and clitoris. Women of all ages should be familiar with the appearance of their genitals and be aware of what is normal for them. In this way, changes that may be the only signs of certain infections or precancerous conditions can be detected early. Early diagnosis means conditions can be diagnosed and treated before they have advanced to later stages. Small sores, ulcers, raw areas, or pigmented areas can be the first and earliest signs of cancer of the vulva. Use a mirror to inspect your vulva monthly to look for these signs.

Women should protect themselves from unwanted pregnancy by using some method of birth control. Ideally, the birth control method should also protect against infections; a barrier method, such as a condom, is ideal. Of course not all methods are perfect, and failures of contraception do occur. Early diagnosis of a missed period allows your maximum choice in expression of your reproductive desires. If you have had sex without birth control or your birth control has failed, ask your doctor about postcoital, or emergency, contraception.

You should have a pelvic examination and a Pap test annually to detect changes in the cervix that could be early signs of cancer (see "The Pap Test"). (See Fig. 1.7A-B) Depending on your situation, your doctor may suggest you have this done more or less often. Any unusual bleeding, pain, or discharge should be brought to the attention of a doctor.

The Pap Test

The Pap test was named after Dr. George Papanicolaou, the physician who developed it. A Pap test can detect changes in the cells on the cervix that could be early signs of cancer. For the test, a women lies on an examining table with her feet in stirrups. An instrument called a speculum is inserted into her vagina to hold it open. With a small brush or scraper, a sample of cells is removed from the cervix and placed on a glass slide so it can be studied under a microscope.

If menstruation starts and is heavy at the time of an appointment, the appointment should be rescheduled. Also, a woman should not douche before the test.

Test results are reported in categories according to the Bethesda system. A negative result means that there are no abnormal cells present in the sample of cells. A positive result means that some abnormal cells are present and may require further testing. As with any test, however, the results depend on the quality of the lab work and the person evaluating the cells.

The Pap test has greatly reduced the number of deaths from cancer of the cervix, and is used to prevent cervical cancer. The test should be performed annually, with a pelvic exam, for women who have been sexually

Figure 1.7 Tests
A woman should have a gynecologic exam, including a Pap smear, at least once a year or more if her doctor advises it. The Pap test (A) is performed by inserting an instrument called a *speculum* into the vagina to hold the walls of the vagina apart. A small spatula or brush is then used to collect a sample of cells from the cervix. The cell sample is then smeared onto a glass slide, which is examined under a microscope. A bimanual pelvic exam (B) is recommended for every woman on a regular basis. For this exam, the doctor feels the shape, size, and position of the internal reproductive organs by inserting two fingers into the vagina and pressing down on the abdomen with the other hand. Many doctors also perform a rectal exam afterward.

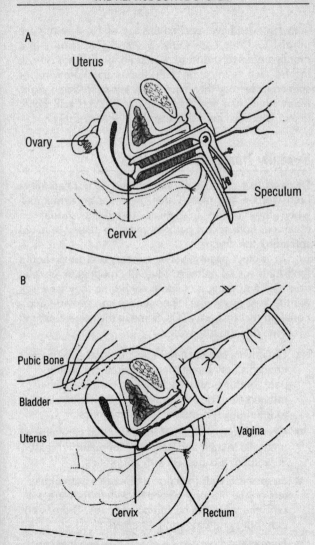

A

Uterus

Ovary

Speculum

Cervix

B

Pubic Bone

Bladder

Uterus

Vagina

Cervix

Rectum

active or who have reached the age of 18. If results are normal for three consecutive years, the woman is in a monogamous relationship or is celibate, and has no risk factors such as infection with human papillomavirus or smoking, she may then have a Pap test every three years. Many physicians feel that a yearly Pap test will better detect abnormal cells that can develop into cancer.

Sexually Transmitted Diseases

Diseases that are sexually transmitted (STDs) can affect both women and men. Often there are no symptoms; when they occur, immediate treatment should be obtained. Both sexual partners must be treated to avoid spreading the disease.

To protect against STDs, women and men should limit their sexual partners. Mutually monogamous relationships and using a condom each time they have sex are the best protection. Spermicides can provide additional protection from STDs. Some of the more common STDs include the following:

- *Chlamydia* is a bacterial infection that can cause urethritis (inflammation of the urethra causing pain, burning, and discharge) in men and pelvic inflammatory disease in women, which can lead to infertility. It is treated with antibiotics.

- *Gonorrhea* is a bacterial infection that can cause urethritis in men and pelvic inflammatory disease in women. It is treated with antibiotics.

- *Herpes* is a viral infection that causes painful blisters on the lips or the genitals. When they are present, the virus can be spread to others. There is no cure but symptoms can be treated.

- *Human papillomavirus* is a viral infection that can cause warts on the external and internal genital area.

In women, it can cause abnormal Pap test results and lead to cancer of the cervix. The warts can be removed but there is no real cure for the virus.

- *Syphilis* is an infection whose first sign is a sore on the genitals that may go away, although the infection does not; it can lead to long-term disability. Syphilis is treated with antibiotics.

- *Trichomonas* is an infection caused by overgrowth of an organism in the vagina, causing a frothy discharge and itching. It is treated with a drug called metronidazole.

Health Care Practitioners

Women can receive care for the reproduction system from any of the following health care professionals:

- Obstetrician-gynecologist: A specialist who has completed 4 years of residency beyond medical school in the field of women's health. This physician may be the woman's primary care doctor or may be consulted for problems relating to the female reproductive system. An obstetrician-gynecologist may receive further training for 2–3 years in a subspecialty: maternal-fetal medicine (high-risk pregnancy and delivery), reproductive endocrinology (hormone and infertility issues), or gynecologic oncology (cancers of the female reproductive organs). Subspecialists are usually located in major medical centers and see patients on referral.

- Internist: A specialist who has completed at least 3 years of internal medicine training beyond medical school. Some internists do gynecological exams (pelvics and Paps) and some do not.

- Family physician: A physician who has completed at least 3 years of specialty training in family practice beyond medical school. Family physicians routinely do gynecological exams.

- Nurse practitioner: A registered nurse who has received additional training and is licensed to perform certain procedures independently.

- Nurse-midwife: A registered nurse who has additional training in providing obstetrical care to women.

SYMPTOMS

Any signs or symptoms of problems in the reproductive system warrant medical attention. In women, problems that can signal a disorder include abnormal bleeding or discharge, pain, or a change in the appearance of the genital organs. In both women and men, any unusual lump or growth that can be felt or seen should receive medical attention.

In young women, any irregular bleeding may be linked to problems with the hormones secreted by the ovaries. In older women, changes in their menstrual periods could signal menopause. Some women may have irregular, unpredictable, and sometimes heavy bleeding during menopause. They have a slightly higher chance of developing precancerous or cancerous changes of the endometrium and should be monitored by a physician. An endometrial biopsy can determine whether precancerous changes are taking place. In this technique, a sample of the tissue lining the uterus is obtained and studied. After menopause, when a woman has stopped having menstrual periods for 12 months, any bleeding should be evaluated.

It is normal for women to have a clear vaginal discharge. This discharge cleans the vagina, maintains its normal state, and keeps it free of organisms. A discharge that is white or yellow, thick or frothy, or has an odor could be a sign of an infection. Itching also may occur. These symptoms could signal a major or minor problem; have them checked so the cause can be identified and treated.

Pain in the pelvic area can occur for many reasons, although it is usually due to either a cramping of the uterus or conditions affecting the ovaries. Pain in the pelvic region also can be related to any of the anatomic structures in this area, including the ureters, bladder, and rectum. If the pain is sudden, severe, and long lasting, or interferes with daily activities, consult your physician.

A pain in your right or left side can be a sign of ovulation. This pain, called *mittelschmerz* (literally, middle pain), is caused by the release of the egg. It may be accompanied by a clear vaginal discharge and increased sex drive. On rare occasions, there may be slight bleeding.

CONDITIONS AND DISORDERS

The female reproductive system is a fairly complicated mechanism that sustains the monthly cycles that are part of fertility as well as pregnancy and childbirth. Because of the complexity of the reproductive organs and the functions needed to maintain it, some normal conditions as well as disorders may require regular medical attention.

Birth Control

Many methods of birth control, or contraception, are available that have a very high degree of safety and effectiveness (see "Contraceptive Failure Rates"). These methods allow you to choose if and when you wish to have children and to plan your family just as you plan other aspects of your life. Without such methods, up to 85 percent of sexually active women using no contraception would be expected to become pregnant in a year. Some methods, such as condoms and spermicides, also provide protection against STDs and cancer of the cervix. All of them allow you control over your reproduction (see "Women's Choices About Contraception").

Hormonal Methods

Pregnancy can be prevented by using hormones to regulate fertility. The hormone estrogen prevents ovulation, the release of an egg. The hormone progesterone blocks the release of the egg during ovulation, although not as well as estrogen, and creates an environment in the uterine lining that makes pregnancy unlikely. These hormones may be used alone or in combination, depending on the technique.

Hormones are used for postcoital, or emergency, contraception, also known as the morning after pill. A doctor or family planning clinic can prescribe the pill, which is usually a combination of birth control pills taken at specific intervals. This technique can be used if a woman has had unprotected intercourse because her method failed or she was sexually assaulted or for any number of reasons. The morning after pill must be administered within hours of intercourse to be effective.

Oral Contraceptives

Birth control pills, or oral contraceptives, are very effective when used properly. There are two types of birth control pills: combination pills, containing the hormones estrogen and progestin, and mini-pills containing only progestin. Progestin is a synthetic version of the natural female hormone progesterone. Women use the

CONTRACEPTIVE FAILURE RATES*

Method	Percentage of Average Use†
Contraceptive implants	0.05%
Vasectomy	0.2
Contraceptive injections	0.4
Tubal sterilization	0.5
IUD	4.0
Pill	6.0
Condom (male)‡	16.0
Cervical cap	18.0
Diaphragm	18.0
Periodic abstinence	19.0
Sponge	24.0
Withdrawal	24.0
Condom (female)‡	26.0
Spermicides	30.0
No method (chance)	85.0

*The failure rate is the estimated percentage of all women using the method who will have an unplanned pregnancy in the first year of use.

†Using a method consistently and correctly—the right way, all the time—makes birth control more effective than these rates show.

‡These methods are most effective against sexually transmitted diseases.

combination pills most often; those women who cannot take estrogen use the mini-pill.

To be effective, the pill must be taken regularly. Some pills are taken daily during a 28-day cycle, whereas others are taken for 21 days, with no pills taken for 7 days before the next pack is started. Missing one pill can result in pregnancy. Birth control pills are generally safe for women in good health who do not smoke. There is no reason to have rest periods from oral contraceptives after they are taken for a number of years.

WOMEN'S CHOICES ABOUT CONTRACEPTION

A woman's choice about which method of birth control to use is largely affected by whether she wishes to have children in the future. Women who do wish to have children choose oral contraceptives most often (49 percent), whereas those who do not plan to have children or who have completed their families choose sterilization (61 percent). About 10 percent of women do not use any form of birth control. These women account for approximately 53 percent of all unintended pregnancies in the United States, half of which end in abortion. Women who are sexually active and not planning to become pregnant should exercise their options of birth control to avoid unintended pregnancy.

Among all women, these are the percentages of women who select specific methods:

Oral contraceptives	27.7%
Tubal sterilization	24.8
Condom	13.1
Periodic abstinence	2.1
IUD	1.8
Spermicides	1.7
Sponge	1

Aside from preventing pregnancy, birth control pills have other benefits. Oral contraceptives protect against cancer of the ovary and the endometrium. The longer a woman takes the pill, the greater the protective effect. Women who take the pill have a lower risk of ovarian cysts, ovarian and endometrial cancer, uterine fibroids, noncancerous breast disease, and ectopic pregnancies. They also tend to have more regular periods with less monthly flow and fewer premenstrual symptoms. The estrogen in oral contraceptives also appears to increase bone density, reducing the risk of bone loss that occurs during menopause.

On the other hand, oral contraceptives have been linked to certain types of cardiovascular disease and cancer of the breast. These effects were observed when higher dose formulations were in use and other factors linked to disease, such as smoking, were not taken into consideration. In general, today's low-dose pills do not seem to pose the same risk. There is, however, an increased risk of thromboembolism (blood clots) in women who smoke and take the pill. Although one study has shown a link between breast cancer and oral contraceptives, others have not been able to confirm that finding.

Oral contraceptives can be used by most healthy women. Do not take birth control pills, however, if any of the following factors apply to you:

- Age over 35 and smoke
- History of vascular disease (including stroke and thromboembolism)
- Uncontrolled high blood pressure, diabetes with vascular disease, high cholesterol
- Active liver disease
- Cancer of the endometrium or breast

Women over age 35 who do not smoke can continue to take a low-dose pill with safety until menopause. Some women may develop bloating, spotting, severe mood swings, or breast tenderness. These problems, or a tendency toward them, require that the woman and her physician work together to find the right formula for her.

Implants
Implants involve a new technique of inserting small plastic tubes containing a progestin or levonorgestrel

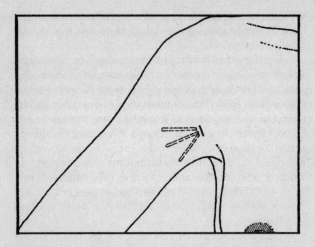

Figure 1.8 Implants
One of the newer methods of birth control is hormonal implants. These small, matchstick-sized tubes are inserted just beneath the surface of the skin, usually on the inner part of a woman's upper arm. The implants contain progestin, a synthetic form of the hormone progesterone, which is slowly released into the bloodstream to prevent pregnancy. Insertion can be done during an office visit, and the implants are effective for up to 5 years.

just under the skin of the arm (see Fig. 1.8). After an injection of local anesthetic to numb the area, the small tubes are imbedded under the skin in the upper arm during an office visit. The hormone is slowly released over a 5-year period. This method of contraception is very effective, but it can cause irregular bleeding and spotting. Other side effects include weight gain, headache, acne, depression, abnormal hair growth, anxiety, and ovarian cysts. The implants need to be surgically removed, and there have been reports that this sometimes can be difficult.

Injections

The injection technique involves injecting a long-acting type of progesterone into the body every 3 months; the failure rate is low. The side effects with this technique include abdominal discomfort, nervousness, dizziness, decreased sex drive, depression, and acne. Some women have weight gain. This method can disrupt menstrual cycles and cause episodes of bleeding and spotting.

Barrier Methods

Some, but not all, barrier methods provide protection against STDs. They can be used in combination to offer extra protection against pregnancy and STDs.

Diaphragm

The diaphragm is a reusable round rubber disk with a flexible rim that fits inside the vagina to cover the cervix (see Fig. 1.9). It should be coated with a spermicide before it is inserted into the vagina. The success of the diaphragm depends partly on spermicidal cream or jelly and partly on its function as a barrier to block entry of the sperm into the cervix. It must be fitted to the shape of the woman's vagina by a doctor or nurse.

The diaphragm should be inserted 1 hour before intercourse and should be left in place at least 6 hours after having sex. If intercourse is repeated, additional spermicide should be inserted into the vagina. When irritation occurs, it may be due to either the rubber or the spermicide. Changing brands of spermicide may solve this problem.

Cervical Cap

The cervical cap is similar to the diaphragm, although it is smaller. Fitting snugly over the cervix, it is held in place by suction (see Fig. 1.10). The cervical cap comes in four sizes to fit a woman's cervix. The cervical

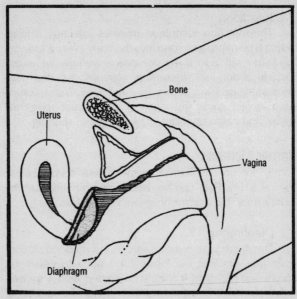

Figure 1.9 Diaphragm
One of the so-called barrier methods of contraception is the diaphragm, a rubber, dome-shaped device that is used with spermicide. It is inserted into the vagina to hold the spermicide in place against the cervix. The flexible rim of the diaphragm helps to hold it in place behind the pubic bone.

cap can be difficult to insert, and it doesn't fit all women. It can be left in a longer time than a diaphragm and can be used to contain menstrual fluid.

Condom

Condoms, for use by both men and women, are all available without prescription. They offer good protection against STDs, including the HIV infection that causes AIDS, as well as pregnancy when used properly. Condoms protect against both viral and bacterial infections, and their use lowers the risk of cancer of the cervix. With new sexual partners of unknown risk for STD, use condoms regardless of other contraceptive methods you may be using. Condoms are disposable. Use one time only and then discard.

The male condom is a sheath that fits over the erect penis and collects the sperm when a man ejaculates. Most condoms are made of latex rubber, although they can be made of animal intestines. Only latex rubber condoms protect against disease, however. Some condoms contain a spermicide (e.g., nonoxynol) that immobilizes and kills the sperm, providing additional contraception. You can get extra protection by using a foam that contains spermicide, along with the condom.

The *male condom* should be applied just before

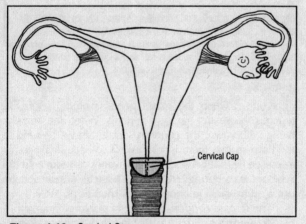

Figure 1.10   Cervical Cap
Similar to the diaphragm, the cervical cap is a small, cup-shaped, rubber device. Also used with spermicide, it is inserted into the vagina and pushed onto the cervix, where it is held in place by suction. The cap is somewhat more difficult to learn to place correctly than the diaphragm, but many women like it because it can be left in place longer and, for some, may be more comfortable.

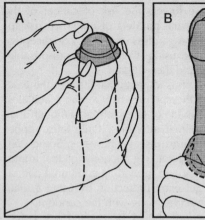
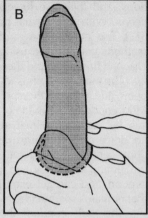

Figure 1.11   Male Condom
The male condom is one of the most widely used forms of contraception. It also offers protection against sexually transmitted diseases, including HIV, the virus that causes AIDS. The rolled-up
condom is placed over the man's erect penis (A) and then unrolled
downward (B). A small space is left at the tip of the condom to
catch the man's semen during ejaculation.

intercourse, when the man's penis is erect, before he
touches the sexual partner's genitals. When the penis is
being withdrawn, the condom should always be held at
the base so that there is less risk of spillage, leakage, or
tears (see Fig. 1.11 A and B). Effectiveness is reduced if the
condom tears during intercourse. If a leak or tear occurs,
use a spermicidal jelly or foam as soon as possible.

The *female condom* is made of polyurethane, a thin
but strong material that resists tearing during use. It consists of two flexible rings connected by a loose-fitting
sheath. One of the rings is used to insert the condom
and hold it inside the vagina. The other ring remains outside and covers the woman's labia and the base of the
penis during intercourse. The female condom is prelu-

bricated and lines the vagina after insertion (see Fig. 1.12). It is designed for one-time use only. One advantage of the female condom is that it can be inserted several hours before sex. Its fairly high failure rate is often due to incorrect use. Used properly, the female condom is nearly as effective as other techniques.

Sponge

The sponge is available without a prescription; it is made of polyurethane and contains a spermicide. Before intercourse, the sponge is inserted into the vagina to cover the cervix, forming both a physical shield and

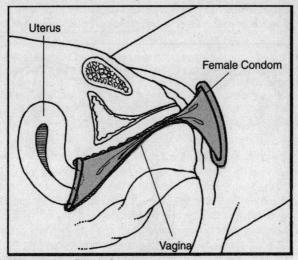

Figure 1.12 Female Condom
The newest form of barrier contraception, the female condom, also offers women protection against sexually transmitted diseases. It consists of a long rubber sheath with a closed ring at one end and a slightly larger, open ring at the other. The closed end is inserted into the vagina and fits over the cervix, like the diaphragm. The open end hangs outside the vagina, so that the interior of the vagina and the cervix are covered.

chemical barrier to sperm. It should be left in place for at least 6 hours after intercourse. The sponge may be left in place up to 24 hours, and it is effective if intercourse is repeated during that time. As with diaphragms or condoms that contain spermicide, a small percentage of users may experience irritation or allergic reactions.

Intrauterine Devices
There are currently two types of intrauterine devices (IUD) available. One is a plastic device shaped like the letter *T* that is wound with copper, and the other is a device that releases the hormone progesterone. When placed inside the uterus, the IUD causes an inflammatory reaction in the uterine lining that prevents pregnancy.

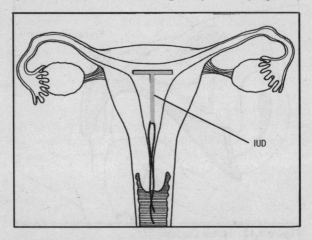

IUD

Figure 1.13 IUD
The intrauterine device (IUD) is a small, plastic device that is inserted into the uterus and left in place to prevent pregnancy. The two forms of IUD currently available are a T-shaped device wound with fine copper wire (shown here) and one containing the hormone progesterone.

The IUD device must be put in place by a trained physician or nurse. It is inserted through the cervix into the uterus. Threads hang through the cervix and must be checked monthly after each period to be sure the IUD is still in place (see Fig. 1.13). The IUD containing progesterone should be replaced every year, while the copper-containing IUD can be used for 8 years.

Some women have uncomfortable short-term side effects, including cramping and dizziness at the time of insertion; bleeding, cramps, and backache that may continue for a few days after insertion; spotting between periods; and longer and heavier periods during the first few cycles after insertion. Use of a copper IUD increases the amount of blood lost each month, while use of the hormone IUD decreases it. The device can migrate into the muscular wall of the uterus and sometimes tear it, although this is rare.

The copper-releasing IUD increases the risk of developing pelvic inflammatory disease (PID), which can result in infertility, especially in those at risk of PID. These people are not good candidates for an IUD; they include women with multiple sexual partners, those with a history of PID, and women under 25 years of age who have not had children. An IUD is a good choice for women who have completed their families and are in monogamous sexual relationships.

Periodic Abstinence

Also known as natural family planning or the rhythm method, periodic abstinence relies on close observation of a woman's cycle to detect when ovulation occurs. Women using this method note the temperature increase that occurs just before ovulation and the change in cervical mucus from dry to wet and slippery that occurs around the same time. It takes into account the fact that sperm live an average of 5 days in the uterus and that the lifespan of the egg after ovulation is 1–3 days. In general, a couple should not have sexual intercourse 7 days before and 3 days after ovulation. Couples who use this method should obtain detailed instructions about it and follow the plan carefully. If used perfectly, this method can be very effective. It is less effective than other forms of birth control, however, because of the difficulty in predicting exactly when ovulation will occur.

Sterilization

Men and women who no longer wish to have children may choose to undergo sterilization. The technique for women is known as tubal ligation, and the one for men is called vasectomy. The procedure for male sterilization is less risky and less expensive than female sterilization. Sterilization should be considered a permanent form of

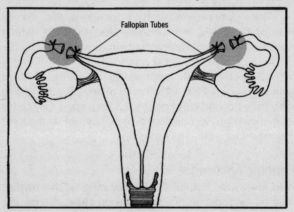

Figure 1.14   Tubal Ligation
Sterilization is a permanent form of birth control. In women, it is done by a procedure called tubal ligation, in which both fallopian tubes are cut and sealed by tying, banding, or clipping the cut ends. The egg released each month by one of the ovaries thus cannot be reached by the man's sperm.

birth control, although in some cases it can be reversed.

Sterilization in women is usually done by laparoscopy. Laparoscopic surgery has been nicknamed Band-Aid surgery because of the small size of the incision near or through the navel.

For the procedure, gas is introduced into the abdominal cavity; the gas pushes the intestine away from the uterus and fallopian tubes. A lighted tube called a laparoscope is inserted through the same incision to allow the surgeon to view the internal area. Operating instruments can either be inserted through the laparoscope or through a second small incision at the pubic hair line. The fallopian tubes are then sealed with electric current that also stops bleeding. In some cases, a ring or clip can be inserted over the tubes through the laparoscope to seal them (see Fig. 1.14). Other reversible means of sealing the tubes are being explored.

The procedure is very effective in preventing pregnancy. Complications are rare but include injuries to the bowel or blood vessels and infection.

Abortion

The medical term for termination of a pregnancy by any cause is *abortion*. The term *spontaneous abortion* describes a natural end of the pregnancy, also called a miscarriage, before the fetus is able to live outside the uterus (about the first 6 months of pregnancy). If a spontaneous abortion is incomplete—if some tissue is retained in the uterus—a medical procedure may be required to be sure the uterus has been emptied and there is no risk of infection. An *elective abortion* refers to the surgical or medical termination of a pregnancy. When a woman is ill and cannot withstand the strain of the pregnancy, termination may be called therapeutic abortion.

With any form of abortion, the initial step is confirming the pregnancy. Most commercially available pregnancy tests inform you of your pregnancy status at the time of the first missed menstrual period. Although this usually occurs about 2 weeks after conception, some women have a lighter period and are unaware they are pregnant until they miss the next period, approximately 6 weeks after the date of conception.

Elective abortions can be performed in a physician's office as early as 1–2 weeks after a missed menstrual period. Using the menstrual extraction technique, the contents of the uterus are removed with a syringe. After 7 weeks of pregnancy, doctors use a procedure called vacuum curettage, the most common method of abortion in the United States. Beyond 13 weeks of pregnancy, more involved procedures are required.

Before the procedure, a woman has her blood type checked and a pregnancy test repeated. She is counseled by health care workers about the procedure and given a chance to ask questions. Consent forms must be signed by the patient and may be required from others, depending on state law. In most cases, the patient is also examined to confirm the length of the pregnancy so the physician can determine the best way to perform the procedure.

Vacuum curettage is performed with a local anesthetic, injected into and around the cervix. The cervix is then dilated, or opened, using a series of gradually larger metal rods or a synthetic material that swells. The contents of the uterus are then removed with a suction device. As the uterus contracts to its previous size, some cramping may result. The amount of blood lost is usually small. In most clinics, only about 1 percent of women have complications, such as infection, perforation of the uterus, or bleeding.

Abortions in later stages have a higher risk of complications and should be performed in a hospital or a specialized clinic. They can be done with suction or by administering agents that bring on labor. In some extreme cases, surgery may be required.

A drug called mifepristone can induce abortion; it is also known as the French pill, or RU–486 and is not currently available in this country. Efforts are ongoing to have this drug available so it can be offered as a safer, nonsurgical approach to abortion.

In the days when abortions were outlawed, women sought abortions from unlicensed providers who frequently did not use sterile techniques and who did not monitor women for complications. As a result, women developed advanced infections that spread from the uterus to the bloodstream and the abdominal cavity. Such infections could result in permanent sterility or death. Today, abortions are extremely safe when performed in a proper medical setting by a licensed practitioner. An abortion has no effect on a woman's ability to have children in the future.

Cancer Detection

When cancer develops in a woman's reproductive organs, it is rarely accompanied by symptoms. (See Fig. 1.15) In some cases, cancer can be prevented by detecting precancerous changes in the cells. In others, noncancerous conditions can cause symptoms that must be explored to rule out cancer. Although the initial evaluation can be done by a gynecologist, a gynecologic oncologist, who specializes in cancer of the reproductive organs, should provide care once cancer is diagnosed. The earlier cancer is detected and treated, the better the chance for cure.

Cervix

The Pap test can detect changes in the cells of the cervix that are not cancer but may warn that cancer could develop (see Fig. 1.7). Some of these changes return to normal on their own, whereas for others, treatment can keep cancer from developing. The Pap test can allow almost all cases of cervical cancer to be prevented, which is why it is so important that you have one regularly.

There are virtually no symptoms during the earliest stage of cervical cancer. The most common early warning signs of cervical cancer are spotting or irregular bleeding or bleeding after intercourse. These signs should prompt an immediate visit to a gynecologist.

Risk factors for cervical cancer include early age at first intercourse, having multiple sexual partners, smoking, and infection with humanpapillomavirus (HPV). Because HPV is spread through sexual contact, the risk factors for contacting this virus include having multiple male sexual partners, who themselves have had multiple sexual partners. Women are most at risk during the teenage years when cervical cells are maturing.

In the Pap test, cells of the cervix are examined under a microscope to detect abnormalities (see Fig. 1.16). The results are reported in categories developed by the National Cancer Institute, called the Bethesda System, and treated accordingly:

- Normal: No abnormal cells are present.
- Atypical Squamous Cells of Undetermined Significance (ASCUS): These cells appear abnormal, but it is not clear exactly what that may mean. Although some doctors may believe that further testing is needed, in most cases these changes can be assessed by a repeat Pap test at a 3–6 month interval, preferably not during menstruation. If results are normal in two consecutive

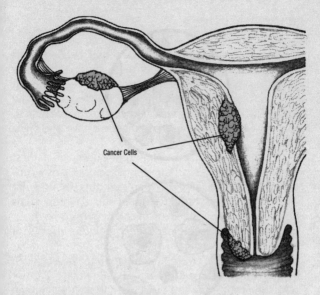

Figure 1.15 Cancer
Possible sites of cancer in women include the ovary, uterus, and cervix.

tests, annual Pap tests can be resumed and no further treatment is needed. About 70 percent of patients with results in this category need no further treatment.

- Low-Grade Squamous Intraepithelial Lesions: Includes changes seen with HPV infection as well as early precancerous changes, also called mild dysplasia or cervical intraepithelial neoplasia grade 1 (CIN 1). About 60 percent of these changes go away on their own, and about 15 percent go on to a more advanced stage. Follow-up may involve monitoring the condition with Pap tests at 3–6-month intervals and performing a pro-

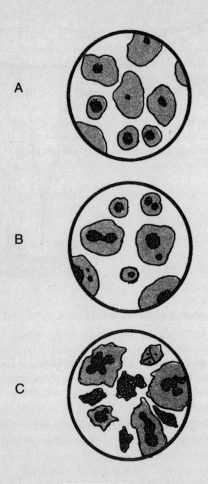

Figure 1.16   Pap Test
In the Pap test, cells collected from the cervix are examined under
a microscope to detect abnormalities. Shown here are normal cervical cells (A), cells showing cervical dysplasia (B), and typical cancer cells (C).

cedure called colposcopy (see "Procedures") if the condition persists.

■ High-Grade Squamous Intraepithelial Lesions: Includes moderate and severe dysplasia (CIN 2 and 3) as well as carcinoma in situ, which is a severe form of precancer. A sample of the tissue is obtained by biopsying the most severe area to confirm the types of abnormalities seen through the colposcope. The affected areas are then removed with local surgery using various techniques: loop electrosurgical excision procedure (LEEP), laser, freezing techniques, or electrosurgery (see "Procedures"). A procedure called cervical conization may be performed to remove a cone-shaped wedge from the cervix.

■ Invasive Cancer: Early stage invasive cancer can be treated with either radical hysterectomy (removal of the uterus) or radiation therapy. In later stages, especially when the lymph nodes are involved, a combination of surgery, radition, and possibly chemotherapy may be used.

There is a 90 percent likelihood that the treatment for early precancerous changes will completely remove any abnormal tissue. About 10 percent of women have an abnormal Pap smear during that first year after treatment. Treatment of this persistent area has a cure rate of about 90 percent. Thus, there is about a 99 percent cure rate with two treatments. Women who have been treated should continue to have yearly Pap tests, however, even after menopause or hysterectomy.

Uterus

Cancer of the lining of the uterus, the endometrium, is the most common gynecologic cancer. About 31,000 cases occur annually. The survival rate for this cancer is high if the cancer is diagnosed in a very early stage.

The most frequent symptom of endometrial cancer is spotting or irregular bleeding, which should alert a woman to seek treatment. Women in the menopausal years should consult their physicians immediately if they develop spotting after their regular periods have stopped for 1 year or more.

The greatest risk factor for endometrial cancer appears to be excess amounts of the hormone estrogen. Estrogen stimulates the uterine lining to grow, causing a condition called endometrial hyperplasia, a form of precancer. The excess estrogen can come from a variety of sources:

- Hormone replacement therapy taken during and after menopause includes estrogen and progesterone. If estrogen is taken alone, a woman's risk of developing endometrial cancer is increased. By taking both estrogen and progesterone pills, however, a woman's risk of cancer is even lower than those who take no therapy.

- Fat cells are the most abundant source of excess estrogen production. Some fat cells normally convert inactive adrenal hormones into very active

---

STAGING OF ENDOMETRIAL CANCER

Stage I	Cancer confined to the body of the uterus.
Stage II	Cancer extended from the body of the uterus to the cervix.
Stage III	Cancer spread out to lymph nodes or onto the ovaries.
Stage IV	Distant spread to the lung or into the bladder or rectum.

estrogenlike hormones. These hormones overstimulate the uterine lining to grow, possibly out of control, into cancer. Women who are slightly overweight have a 3-fold risk of developing endometrial cancer and those who are nearly twice their recommended weight have a 10-fold risk of developing endometrial cancer.

The diagnosis is confirmed by performing a uterine biopsy to obtain a sample of the lining to study. This procedure can be performed in a physician's office, without any anesthesia. The "D&C," or dilation and curettage, is rarely needed now that suction biopsies can be done in the office.

Treatment usually consists of a hysterectomy. The ovaries are usually removed (oophorectomy), along with the lymph nodes. A careful search is made for any sign of further spread (see "Staging of Endometrial Cancer"). A general gynecologist can perform the surgery in early stage cancer but a gynecologic oncologist should always be available if advanced disease is found during the surgery. If advanced disease is diagnosed preoperatively, the gynecologic oncologist should perform the surgery. After surgery and complete pathological evaluation of the uterus, the ovaries, and the lymph nodes, further treatment may be recommended in the form of either radiation or chemotherapy.

Ovarian Cancer

Ovarian cancer is the most malignant of all of the gynecologic cancers. Approximately 24,000 women develop ovarian cancer each year, and unfortunately many are not diagnosed until the cancer is in advanced stages. The risk factors for ovarian cancer include advanced age, not having children or having them late in life, and a family history of ovarian cancer or other cancers such as breast or colon cancers.

Ovarian cancer gives only vague early warning signs, such as a change in bowel pattern, a feeling of bloating, or simply pelvic discomfort. These symptoms may be due to pressure from a pelvic mass or tumor implants on the bowel wall.

When ovarian cancer grows, some women think they are only getting fat and don't investigate the cause of the swelling. The cancer can cause fluid to accumulate within the abdominal cavity, causing the abdomen to swell. This fluid contains cancer cells and can spread even into the lung cavity, where more fluid can accumulate.

Since there are so few warning signs in the early stages, this cancer is usually diagnosed later, when tumor nodules from the ovaries extend to the surface of the liver, the bowel, the stomach, or inside the abdominal wall. Cancer is often suspected by pelvic exam and confirmed by ultrasound. A blood test also can be performed to measure a substance called CA–125 that circulates in the blood. CA–125 is used as a tumor marker because levels are increased when tumors are present. Because levels are increased by the presence of many other benign disorders, this test is not used to screen healthy women.

Therapy usually begins with surgery to remove all the tumor, followed by chemotherapy. The chemotherapy is fairly effective at removing any tumor cells left after surgery. While a complete cure of this cancer occurs in only about 20–30 percent of women, chemotherapy usually prolongs life very significantly.

Ovarian Cysts

Often a cyst may develop on an ovary. This fluid-filled growth is not cancerous in most cases. Some may be the earliest sign that a cancer has formed, however, so all ovarian cysts should be taken seriously and evaluated. Ovarian cysts may have no symptoms; large cysts can cause a feeling of pelvic pressure or fullness. Diagnosis is usually by vaginal ultrasound: A small probe is passed into the vagina that reveals details of the ovaries and uterus. The CA-125 blood test can also be performed to assess the likelihood of ovarian cancer. Treatment of ovarian cysts range from careful monitoring of simple small cysts to surgical removal of any ovarian cysts that may suggest a malignancy. Oral contraceptives do not make an ovarian cyst disappear any faster. If you have an ovarian cyst that is under observation, your doctor should check it again within three months to make sure it has not changed or grown larger. Always get a second opinion before having surgery for an ovarian cyst.

Vagina

Cancer of the vagina that does not involve the vulva or the cervix is rare. One form is caused by exposure to a drug called diethylstilbestrol, or DES, in women whose mothers took the drug while they were pregnant. In the early 1950s DES was prescribed to women who were at risk of losing their pregnancies. Now, their daughters are at risk for some cancers of the vagina. A registry has been created to keep track of these women so they can receive careful monitoring. The cancer usually develops around age 19; treatment is by hysterectomy, and it has a 90 percent cure rate if identified in the earliest stage of growth.

Vulva

Vulvar cancer is a rare gynecologic malignancy. It almost always strikes women who are in the menopausal years and appears to be linked to infection with HPV. The cancer appears as a small sore or small lump on one of the outer lips of the vulva. Sometimes it can itch, but it usually does not cause any pain. Many women delay seeing their gynecologists, hoping the sore will disappear; however, this delay allows for continued tumor growth. If you have a small sore, lump, or ulcer on any area of the vulva that is new and does not go away within a week, see your physician.

The diagnosis is based on the results of a biopsy, in which the area is numbed and a small amount of tissue is removed to be studied. If the cancer is found in early stages, surgery is performed. Usually, the area of cancer must be removed with a rim of normal tissue of approximately 1 inch in diameter all the way around the cancer. This is called a radical partial vulvectomy. In most stages of disease, lymph nodes in the groin should also be removed. If cancer has spread to the lymph nodes, radiation therapy is usually required.

Ectopic Pregnancy

Normally, once the egg is fertilized in the fallopian tubes, it travels to the uterus and becomes implanted there. When, for any reason, the fertilized egg implants anywhere else along the route, the pregnancy is said to be ectopic, or in the wrong place (see Fig. 1.17).

Ectopic pregnancy occurs when the opening of the fallopian tube is twisted or narrowed, due to scar tissue formed by infection or surgery. The passage of the fertilized egg to the uterus is blocked, and the egg begins to develop within the fallopian tube lining, on the surface of the ovary, or within the abdominal or pelvic cavity. The egg can only develop for a few weeks before its growth is hindered by the size of the fallopian tube.

In an ectopic pregnancy, symptoms of early pregnancy, an abnormally light period, and pelvic pain can occur. Many women have no symptoms until the pregnancy causes a rupture of the fallopian tube or there is bleeding from a nearby blood vessel. This causes severe abdominal pain, shock, and collapse—a medical emergency of the first order.

If you have a history of tubal infections or previous ectopic pregnancy and suspect you are pregnant, you should be carefully monitored by your physician to be sure that the pregnancy is within the uterus. Ectopic pregnancy is diagnosed by doing tests to measure hormone levels that indicate pregnancy. Once pregnancy has been confirmed, ultrasound can determine its location and size.

If the fallopian tube has ruptured, ectopic pregnancy is an emergency that requires surgery to remove the pregnancy and control bleeding. In some cases, the tube can then be rejoined. Many surgeons are now performing this procedure through the laparoscope. Conservative surgery in which the fallopian tube is simply opened and the pregnancy lifted out is frequently possible and conserves the tube, and thus your ability to have children. Another procedure for small, early ectopic

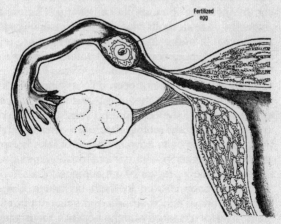

Fertilized egg

Figure 1.17 Ectopic Pregnancy
In an ectopic pregnancy, the fertilized ovum becomes attached in a place other than inside the uterus. Most ectopic pregnancies occur in a fallopian tube.

pregnancies involves the intramuscular injection of chemotherapy; the usual result is loss of the pregnancy in about 7 days.

Endometriosis

The tissue that lines the inside of the uterus responds to hormones that cause it to thicken and bleed each month. This tissue can also grow outside the uterus, on the pelvic organs. When this occurs, these areas can become inflamed and sometimes painful, and scar tissue develops.

Some women with endometriosis, even severe endometriosis, have no symptoms. Others can have intense pain, especially when the endometrial tissue is shed into the pelvic area during the menstrual period. The pain can be felt throughout the entire area or may be confined to the uterus. Pain usually appears only during the menstrual period, but can start just before and gradually increase until bleeding starts, usually easing after up to 72 hours. In addition to pelvic pain, endometriosis is a common cause of infertility because it causes the fallopian tubes to malfunction.

Researchers have not been able to pinpoint causes of endometriosis. One theory is that endometrial tissue travels through the fallopian tubes and becomes implanted on surrounding structures (see Fig. 1.18). Delay of pregnancy to beyond age 30 or later is associated with a higher risk of endometriosis. Women who have never had a pregnancy are at highest risk.

Laparoscopy is used for both definitive diagnosis and treatment of endometriosis. The treatment of endometriosis depends largely on the patient's needs and desires. If relief of pain is of most importance and childbearing has been completed, a hysterectomy with removal of the ovaries, followed by hormone replacement therapy, is often recommended. When fertility is desired, the spots of endometriosis can be removed by laparoscopy with laser therapy. Unfortunately, the condition recurs in about one-third of women treated.

Synthetic hormones can be used to shrink the endometriosis implants, but the effect is temporary. The implants usually return to their premedication level within a few months after treatment ends. Treatment can be given for only 6 months because it decreases the estrogen level. This brief remission of the disease can be time enough to allow conception soon after, if that is desired. Because prevention of ovulation can reduce the discomfort, many women take oral contraceptives.

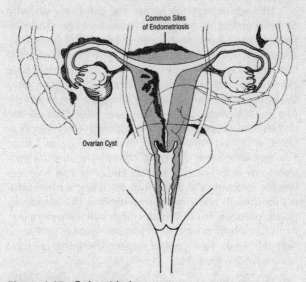

Figure 1.18   Endometriosis
Endometriosis is a condition in which tissue similar to that lining the uterus is present outside the uterus. It may be attached to the outside of the uterus, ovaries, or tubes, or it may be present in other areas of the abdomen.

However, some still have pain and require surgery for relief.

Fibroids

Benign fibrous growths of the uterine wall are called fibroids. Some fibroids bulge outward from the wall; others extend from the uterine surface on a stalk. A fibroid can also extend into the uterine lining, compressing the endometrium or forming a growth on a stem within the endometrial cavity. About 20 percent of women of reproductive age have fibroids, and for most of them the fibroids pose no problem.

Fibroids enlarge the uterus and can cause pressure and discomfort in the pelvis, however. Internal uterine fibroids can also compress the endometrial lining and cause excessive bleeding during and occasionally between menstrual periods. Younger women rarely have fibroids, but when they do, the fibroids can press against the lining of the uterus causing infertility. The most serious complication is pressure and blockage of the ureters, the tubes draining the kidneys. On rare occasions, a fibroid can develop into a malignant tumor. Fibroids have been the most common reason for hysterectomy in the past, as well as currently. The only reason for removing the fibroids or for doing a hysterectomy for fibroids is if they cause symptoms like bladder or pelvic pressure, excessive bleeding, infertility, or pain.

Ultrasound is used to determine the size and location of fibroids. Two types of surgery, if needed, are used to remove the growths:

- Hysterectomy to remove the uterus and with it, the fibroids
- Myomectomy to remove the fibroids only, leaving the uterus intact

The selection of the type of surgery used rests with the woman and her surgeon. For a woman who wants to maintain her fertility, a myomectomy is the treatment of choice. It might also be preferred by the woman who wishes to have her uterus and ovaries left intact.

Myomectomy usually involves more blood loss than a hysterectomy, because the fibroid can have a rich blood supply. During a hysterectomy, the location of each blood vessel that feeds the uterus is well known and can be clamped off so that little bleeding occurs. During myomectomy, the blood supply to the fibroid is less clearly defined and blood loss can be heavy. Many gynecologists recommend that women who do not want to retain fertility simply have the top half or the entire uterus removed in what is called a partial hysterectomy.

Sometimes this procedure can be made easier by shrinking the fibroid prior to surgery. This is done by pre-scribing hormones that mimic menopause and decrease the amount of estrogens, resulting in shrinkage of the fibroid by as much as 50 percent.

Women can usually become pregnant after removal of a fibroid and carry the pregnancy to full term, although they may occasionally require a caesarean delivery.

Menopause

At menopause, a woman stops menstruating and her ovaries no longer produce estrogen. The average age at the last menstrual period is 51. This natural process begins several years before, as a woman's ovaries produce less and less estrogen. The lack of estrogen can produce a number of effects:

- Hot flashes or flushes can occur. These are sudden feelings of heat that spread over the body, often accompanied by a flushed face and sweating. They appear at any time without warning and are most troublesome at night when they can interfere with sleep.

- Vaginal tissues may become dryer, thinner, and less flexible. This can result in painful intercourse, urinary tract problems, or sagging of pelvic organs because the tissues that support them lose their elasticity.

- Osteoporosis, or bone loss can cause bones to become thin and brittle. Supplemental estrogen can help guard against it, as can a diet high in calcium, regular exercise, and stopping smoking.

- Cardiovascular disease becomes more of a risk for women after menopause because estrogen no longer gives them natural protection from heart attack and stroke.

- Emotional changes, such as mood swings, irritability, and depression can accompany menopause, but these symptoms are more likely related to insomnia caused by hot flashes at night than to the lack of estrogen.

Not all women have all of these symptoms and they are not always long lasting. You can continue to have a full and healthy life for many years beyond menopause. Some of the symptoms of menopause can be eased through diet and exercise. Others can be relieved by replacing the estrogen no longer produced by the ovaries. Hormone replacement therapy can relieve the symptoms of menopause, in addition to lowering the risk of heart disease and osteoporosis.

Estrogen is given along with the hormone progestin (a synthetic version of the natural hormone progesterone) to protect against endometrial cancer, a risk when estrogen is taken alone. Estrogen by itself causes the lining of the uterus to overgrow and increases the risk of cancer of the endometrium. Progestin is taken with estrogen to oppose it and keep the lining of the endometrium in check. In fact, taking progestin with estrogen actually lowers the risk of cancer to less than that of a woman not taking hormone therapy.

Estrogen is processed through the liver and affects the levels of cholesterol. Estrogen increases high-density cholesterol (the good cholesterol) and lowers low-density cholesterol (the bad cholesterol), thus reducing the risk of heart disease. Without estrogen, a woman's risk of heart disease approaches that of a man by age 65.

Women are at higher risk of osteoporosis because they have less bone mass than men to begin with and because they tend to have less calcium stored in their bones. Thus, when they lose the protective effect of estrogen, the natural process of bone loss speeds up so they are losing bone faster than it is being replaced.

Osteoporosis and cardiovascular disease do not have symptoms in their early stages as they are conditions that develop over time. Hormone replacement therapy to prevent symptoms of menopause also helps prevent these conditions. To provide long-term protection, the therapy must be taken long term.

Hormone replacement therapy is not for everyone. It is not recommended for women who have had breast cancer, endometrial cancer, or liver cancer. The link between breast cancer and hormone replacement therapy is still not clear. There may be a slight increase in a woman's chance of developing breast cancer if she has been taking hormones for more than 15 years.

Hormone replacement therapy can have other side effects. The progestin causes monthly bleeding or spotting, which can be unexpected and bothersome. Other side effects include breast tenderness, fluid retention, swelling, mood changes, and pelvic cramping. Because of the side effects, some women choose to take estrogen alone. These women should be monitored carefully for abnormal bleeding. Their doctors may suggest that an endometrial biopsy be performed so a small amount of tissue can be examined.

Women who prefer not to take hormone replacement therapy can obtain relief of symptoms and help prevent bone loss and heart disease in other ways. To facilitate decisions about hormones, women should have a fasting cholesterol and a bone density test. Estrogen cream, used in the vagina, can treat vaginal dryness. A balanced diet rich in calcium and low in fat, regular exercise, and avoiding alcohol and tobacco can help reduce the rate of bone loss and protect against heart disease. Regardless of age or whether they are taking hormone replacement therapy, women should continue to have regular pelvic exams, mammograms, and Pap tests after they reach menopause.

Menstrual Problems

Most women experience some discomfort with their menstrual periods. Certain conditions, such as endometriosis or fibroids, can increase pain during menstrual periods. Any severe pain, unusual spotting or bleeding, or missed menstrual periods could be a sign of a problem that requires medical attention.

Amenorrhea
Amenorrhea is the absence of menstruation. This absence is normal before puberty, after menopause, and during pregnancy. Primary amenorrhea occurs when a woman reaches the age of 18 and has never had a period. It is usually caused by a problem in the endocrine system that regulates hormones. Secondary amenorrhea is present when a woman has had regular periods that

stop for longer than 12 months. Amenorrhea may be triggered by a wide range of events:

Primary amenorrhea

■ Ovarian failure
■ Problems in the nervous system or the pituitary gland in the endocrine system that affect maturation at puberty
■ Birth defects in which the reproductive structures do not develop properly

Secondary amenorrhea

■ Problems that affect estrogen levels, such as stress, weight loss, exercise, or illness
■ Problems affecting the pituitary, thyroid, or adrenal gland
■ Ovarian tumors or surgical removal of the ovaries

To diagnose and treat amenorrhea it may be necessary to consult a reproductive endocrinologist. Treatment is based on the problem diagnosed. Blood tests are usually performed and many patients are asked to keep a record of their early morning temperatures to detect the rise in temperature that occurs with ovulation.

Cramps

The sensation of spasmodic cramping or a feeling of chronic achy fullness can occur with a normal menstrual cycle and a normal anatomy. The pain is due to uterine contractions, caused by substances called prostaglandins.

Prostaglandins circulate within the blood. They can cause diarrhea by speeding up the contractions of the intestinal tract and lower blood pressure by relaxing the muscles of blood vessels. Thus many women frequently notice that severe menstrual pain is associated with mild diarrhea and occasionally an overall sensation of faintness in which they become pale, sweaty, and sometimes nauseated. Some women actually have fainting spells because of the low blood pressure resulting from the action of prostaglandins.

To relieve cramps, your doctor may recommend drugs called prostaglandin inhibitors or nonsteroidal anti-inflammatory drugs (NSAIDs), which are available without a prescription. Taking medication immediately at the onset of any symptoms usually results in dramatic improvement or complete relief. Taking these drugs even before symptoms begin may help, too. Relief also may be obtained by applications of heat and mild exercise.

Excessive Bleeding

Some women experience a menopause characterized by irregular, unpredictable, often heavy bleeding. If you develop severe irregular bleeding as you approach menopause, or experience new bleeding a year after your final period, your doctor should do a biopsy to confirm that no precancerous changes have taken place. This biopsy does not need to be the traditional dilation and curettage (D&C) that is performed in a hospital under general anesthesia. Rather, the biopsy is a simple procedure that takes place in the doctor's office. A slender, soft, plastic canula is inserted through the cervix and a small sample of uterine tissue is obtained. The cost of this biopsy is about 10 percent of the cost of a regular D&C and provides the same information. These tests are 99.5 percent reliable in diagnosing a precancerous condition or cancer, if present. If there is no sign of cancer, excessive bleeding can be treated with hormone therapy or surgery on the lining of the uterus.

Pelvic Inflammatory Disease

Infection with the STDs chlamydia and gonorrhea can lead to pelvic inflammatory disease (PID). In PID, infection spreads upward through the cervix, the uterus, and the fallopian tubes into the pelvic cavity. White blood cells battling the infection cause a puslike discharge to surround the ovaries. The body tries to wall off this infection by creating filmy adhesions (a fibrous wall) from organ to organ to limit the spread of the infection. The adhesions can distort the fallopian tubes and result in infertility.

Early symptoms of PID include pelvic pain associated with fever and weakness; there also may be a vaginal discharge. If the infection continues, an abscess can form within the pelvis. The typical PID attack strikes after a menstrual period and begins with pelvic pain. Motion, even walking, can be painful. If the abscess develops, it can send bacteria into the bloodstream, causing high fever, chills, joint infections, and even death.

Diagnosis usually is based on the symptoms and presence of the abscess. In some cases, a sample of the discharge from the abscess can be used to identify the organism causing the infection. Antibiotics can stop the infection before an abscess has formed, if treatment is started early. If the infection is severe, some patients may require intravenous antibiotics in a hospital setting. Surgery may be necessary to drain an abscess, but it is usually not necessary to remove the uterus, tubes, and ovaries.

Premenstrual Syndrome

The regular, recurring symptoms that occur just prior to menstruation are called premenstrual syndrome (PMS). PMS is not a disease but rather a collection of symptoms that disappear once the menstrual period has begun.

Nearly all menstruating women experience a set of symptoms that tell them their periods are coming. For some women, these symptoms can be quite severe, involving a combination of emotional and physical changes. Emotional changes may include anger, anxiety, confusion, mood swings, tension, crying, depression, and an inability to concentrate. Physical symptoms include bloating, swollen breasts, fatigue, constipation, headache, and clumsiness.

The diagnosis rests on confirming the cyclic nature of these symptoms and ruling out any underlying psychological or physical dysfunction. Many women are asked to chart their symptoms so they can be related to the menstrual cycle to detect a pattern. The symptoms usually occur about 7 days before a menstrual period and go away once it begins.

The cause of PMS is unknown, despite extensive research into abnormal types of hormones that are secreted at this time, unusual ratios of one hormone to another, and imbalance between sodium and body water retention. Many theories have been studied, but none has been shown to be the primary cause. As a result, the condition is difficult to treat.

Treatment is generally aimed at relieving symptoms. Keeping a calendar and being aware of when symptoms occur helps most women; simply knowing their distressing symptoms are related to the onset of their periods can have a calming effect. There are other things you can try to ease symptoms of PMS:

- Dietary changes provide relief for some women: decreasing sodium, sugar, caffeine, and alcohol; increasing complex carbohydrates; and eating smaller, more frequent meals.

- Dietary supplementation of calcium, magnesium, and vitamins B_6 and E may reduce symptoms.

- Exercise has been shown to help in depression and, theoretically, may be of some benefit for PMS.

- Diuretics can relieve the feeling of bloating and swelling caused by fluid retention.

- Pain can be relieved with nonsteroidal anti-inflammatory drugs (NSAIDs).

- Oral contraceptives are helpful in relieving symptoms in some women.

- Severe breast tenderness can be relieved by taking bromocriptine, a drug that stops the production of certain hormones, but this drug does not help other PMS symptoms.

Many medications have been tried with limited success. Some of them are expensive and most have side effects. It may be necessary to combine some remedies on a trial and error basis, along with modifications in diet and exercise.

Rape

Rape is sexual intercourse by force; it is epidemic in our country. This violent crime has both psychological as well as medical aspects that affect women's health.

A rape should be reported within 48 hours of its occurrence, as crucial evidence of it is more difficult to obtain after that time. Women should not wash, bathe, urinate, defecate, drink, or take any medication prior to reporting a rape. A practitioner experienced in this area should perform a thorough exam so there is evidence available if charges are brought against the accused rapist.

A physician first asks the woman to describe what happened, and then examines her clothing for damage, taking particular note if there are any materials such as soil or stains such as body fluids sticking to the clothing. The physician next asks if any drugs or alcohol were taken by the woman or the rapist, because this may become an important issue during court procedures.

The physical exam consists of looking for evidence on the whole body, even though not every woman who has been raped has been physically injured. The physician measures and charts all injuries and may photograph them, looking carefully for bite marks, bruises, grip marks, and scratches. Samples are taken of the vaginal fluid to check for infection or sperm. Mouth swabs and saliva samples are obtained to look for bacteria and semen and possibly to perform DNA studies of the sample. Urine samples may be obtained to determine whether drugs were involved. Blood samples are obtained to test for HIV as well as hepatitis. If the HIV test is negative, another HIV test should be done in 6 months to determine whether the virus was contracted during the rape. A woman may be given treatment against possible STDs, and she should be offered emergency contraception if there is a chance pregnancy could result from the assault.

After the exam, comfort, support, and counseling are key to complete recovery. There are many groups available to counsel women who are recovering from previous molestation or rape.

Vaginitis

The internal environment of the vagina consists of a delicate balance of organisms that, along with normal vaginal secretions, keep it healthy and clean. When that balance is disrupted by either an infection, a health problem, or some type of irritation, vaginitis can occur. Bacteria or yeast that grows normally in the vagina can overgrow and cause itching, redness, and pain in the vaginal area. Infections from other organisms, as well as allergic reactions, can also cause vaginitis.

Any new discharge accompanied by an odor, or abnormal itching, could be a sign of a vaginal infection. The characteristics of the discharge—its color, odor, and amount—can be a clue to the cause. Yeast is the most common cause of vaginitis, but bacteria and parasites can also cause it. The cause of vaginitis must be identified for treatment to be effective.

Bacterial Vaginosis

Among the more common vaginal infections, bacterial vaginosis is caused by the *Gardnerella, Bacteriodes,* and *Peptostreptococcus* bacteria. The primary symptom is a foul-smelling, profuse, watery vaginal discharge.

The diagnosis is confirmed by microscopic examination of the discharge. Treatment for this infection is the antibiotic metronidazole. Often, the infection recurs; longer treatment may be needed to prevent recurrences.

Yeast Infection

Some women are unusually susceptible to this most common of all vaginal infections. The cause may be a recent course of antibiotics that can decrease the normal vaginal bacteria and allow for an overgrowth of yeast. Other conditions, like diabetes and HIV infection, are also associated with recurrent yeast infections.

Your doctor will want to confirm that yeast is the cause by examining the vaginal discharge under a microscope. Discuss multiple recurrent yeast infections with your physician, because other problems such as diabetes should be ruled out.

Once you can recognize the symptoms of yeast vaginitis, you can treat yourself by purchasing any one of the over-the-counter antifungal creams or suppository preparations. Treatment is also available in pill form by prescription.

PROCEDURES FOR WOMEN

Cryotherapy

Cryotherapy involves freezing cells on the cervix to remove abnormal cells. Freezing kills cells but does not remove them from the vagina. The dead cells dissolve into the vaginal fluid and are washed away in the normal secretions. This can cause an increased vaginal discharge for about 2 weeks after the procedure.

Colposcopy

In colposcopy, the cervix, vagina, and vulva skin are examined systematically under microscopic magnification. When abnormal areas are detected, a sample is taken for further examination (a biopsy).

During the procedure, a speculum is inserted in the vagina to spread the vaginal walls, and a vinegar solution is sprayed into the cervix. The abnormal surface cells appear white, and normal cells remain pink. The entire area is examined, and a biopsy of any white area is performed.

Most women have a slight cramp for a minute or so during the biopsy. Otherwise, this procedure requires no anesthesia and is well tolerated. If a woman has severe cramps with her menstrual cycle, medication can be given before the exam to reduce discomfort.

Occasionally a scraping of tissue is obtained from

the inner lining of the cervix beyond the limits of the area that can be seen. This scraping provides extra assurance that the entire abnormality has been identified. Once the biopsy results are available, therapy can be started.

Dilation and Curettage

Often referred to as a D&C, dilation and curettage removes the lining and contents of the uterus. Once the cervix is widened by dilators, the uterine lining is scraped out with a curette, a spoonlike instrument. A D&C is used to perform abortions, remove the lining of the uterus in cases of severe bleeding, or test for uterine cancer (see Fig. 1.19). A D&C is performed in a hospital or an ambulatory surgery center using general anesthetic. Rapid recovery with minimal spotting for 1 to 2 days can be expected. It has largely been replaced by the office biopsy.

Hysterectomy

A complete or total hysterectomy (see Fig. 1.20A) is removal of the entire uterus with the cervix. A partial hysterectomy involves removing only a portion of the uterus (see Fig. 1.20B). A radical hysterectomy involves the removal of the uterus, cervix, lymph nodes, and other support structures around the cervix and uterus (see Fig. 1.20C). A hysterectomy can be performed through the vagina or through a cut in the abdomen, depending on the reasons for the surgery.

Reasons for performing a hysterectomy should be clearly understood prior to the procedure. Following are the most common reasons for a hysterectomy:

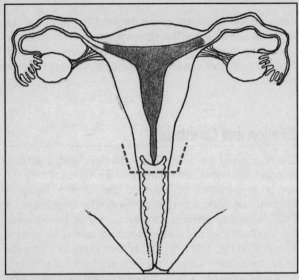

Figure 1.19. Dilation and Curettage
Dilation and curettage (D&C) is a procedure used to remove the endometrium (the lining of the uterus) and the contents of the uterus. A speculum is inserted into the vagina, the cervix is grasped with a small tonguelike instrument, and the inside of the uterus is gently scraped out with another instrument.

- Fibroids
- Endometriosis
- Cancer
- Endometrial hyperplasia
- Menstrual/menopausal symptoms
- Cervical dysplasia
- Pain

A vertical incision in the lower abdomen is used for abdominal hysterectomy or for cancer or a very large fibroid. For other conditions, a horizontal incision is placed just above the pubic bone, which can be hidden in the pubic hair (see Fig. 1.21). This location results in less postoperative pain.

A vaginal hysterectomy involves less discomfort than an abdominal hysterectomy because no abdominal incision must be made. Vaginal hysterectomies are seldom performed on women who have had no children because the ligaments are tighter and the vaginal passage is small. It is indicated when there is a small uterus, and the patient has had children, because the vagina and the connecting structures of the uterus are more pliable.

Vaginal hysterectomy is now available to more women because it can be done with a laparoscope. When the laparoscope is used, it is placed into the abdomen through a small incision in the abdominal wall. The laparoscope is a telescopelike probe that can identify the structures and cut away problems outside the uterus, such as adhesions. The uterus can then be removed through the vagina with less postoperative pain and scarring.

Recovery time varies depending on the procedure. Usually, normal activities, including sex, can be resumed in about 4–6 weeks. Until then, activities such as driving, sports, and light physical work may be increased gradually. Adhesions, or scar tissue, can develop after any surgery. They can cause pain during bowel function, intercourse, or exercise. If adhesions are particularly troublesome, laparoscopic surgery can be used to relieve them, although they may return in the future.

Very few women notice a change in their sexual sensations after hysterectomy that could be related to the functions of the uterus during sexual activity or to their own sense of loss of their uterus. For most women, however, hysterectomy has no effect on sexual satisfaction. Many women have a sense of freedom from symptoms of the condition corrected, as well as from the concern of monthly periods and potential pregnancy. If you

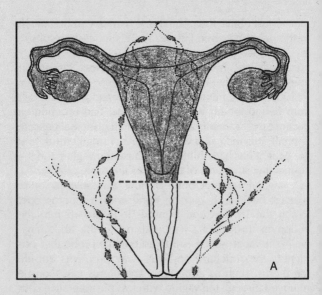

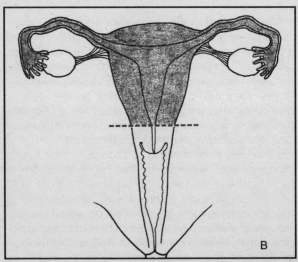

have any doubts about having a hysterectomy, always get a second opinion.

Hysteroscopy

Hysteroscopy allows the inside of the uterus and the openings of the fallopian tubes to be viewed on a video camera or a monitor. The hysteroscope is a telescope that is inserted to look at the walls of the uterus for signs

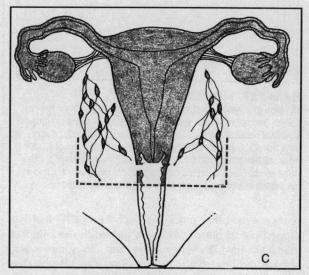

Figure 1.20   Hysterectomy
Hysterectomy, the surgical removal of the uterus, may be done in a number of ways, depending on the problem being treated. A total hysterectomy (A) involves the removal of the entire uterus, along with the ovaries and fallopian tubes. In a partial hysterectomy (B), the uterus and tubes are removed, but the ovaries and cervix are left in place. A radical hysterectomy (C) entails removal of the entire uterus, the tubes, and the ovaries, along with the lymph nodes and the support structures surrounding these organs.

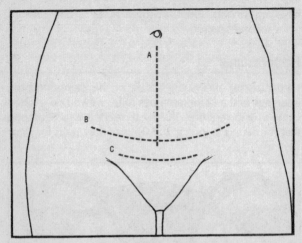

Figure 1.21 Hysterectomy Incisions
The type of incision used for a hysterectomy depends on the reason for and nature of the problem for which it is being performed.
A vertical incision (A) may be used for uterine cancer or a very
large fibroid. Other conditions may necessitate the use of a transverse, or horizontal, incision (B). The location and size of a transverse incision also depends on the problem being treated; a low
transverse incision (C) often can be hidden in the pubic hair.

of disease or other problems (such as an IUD that has
slipped out of place). It can be guided to the fallopian
tubes to find any obstruction and, in some cases,
remove it. Some surgical procedures can also be performed with hysteroscopy. The procedure may be performed in a doctor's office using local anesthetic.

Laparoscopy

In laparoscopy, a lighted tube with a magnifying lens on
the end allows the operator to see inside the body.
Laparoscopy can be used to diagnose a condition, such

as endometriosis; it also can be used to perform surgery.

Laparoscopic surgery uses small holes or punctures rather than one large incision. These small incisions result in less postoperative pain and shorter recovery, as compared with an abdominal incision. Women usually return to work within 3 or 4 days after laparoscopy in comparison to 4 to 6 weeks after more extensive surgery.

Many procedures can now be done through a laparoscope:

- Hysterectomy
- Removal of the gallbladder
- Removal of segments of colon
- Assisting vaginal hysterectomy
- Removal of fibroids
- Removal of the fallopian tubes
- Sterilization
- Removal of ovarian cysts

Laser

Laser therapy uses a beam of very intense and focused light to perform surgery. It is used to remove abnormal tissue from the cervix that could be a sign of early cancer. The laser also can remove warts that result from HPV infection. To increase the likelihood of complete cure, a small margin of normal tissue may also be removed. An anesthetic is given before surgery, and recovery is usually very rapid.

Loop Electrosurgical Excision Procedure

For a loop electrosurgical excision procedure, known as LEEP, a high-intensity electrical current passes through a wire used to cut a thin slice of tissue from the cervix. This tissue can be examined under a microscope. In addition to obtaining samples of tissue for diagnosis, LEEP also can be used for treatment by removing abnormal tissue. A local anesthetic is administered before the procedure, and pain medication may be given to ease postoperative discomfort. A minimal discharge is experienced after this procedure.

Ultrasound

In ultrasound, inaudible super-swift sound waves are projected into the body. The reflected echoes are captured to create an image of the internal structures of the body; this is transferred to a black and white image on a monitor screen. From this image the physician or diagnostic expert can tell the size and shape of the ovaries, the uterus, and other pelvic structures. It can determine the age and exact location of the fetus within the uterus. In some situations physical details of a fetus can be identified; it is especially helpful in confirming a possible multiple birth.

PART II
The Kidneys and the Urinary System

Tamara G. Bavendam, M.D.,
F.A.C.S., and Sandra P. Levison,
M.D., F.A.C.P.

The urinary system eliminates waste products while saving materials needed by the body. It does this by producing and excreting urine, a watery substance made up of excess fluid, waste products, and toxins. The body produces urine continually. No conscious effort is needed to produce urine, but excreting it does require being aware of when the bladder is full and getting to the toilet to urinate.

The urinary system includes the kidneys, the ureters, the bladder, and the urethra. Together, these structures are called the urinary tract.

HOW THE URINARY SYSTEM WORKS

The kidneys are a pair of bean-shaped organs that lie in the upper part of the abdomen, next to the spine at the base of the lower ribs (see Fig. 2.1). Human beings need only one functioning kidney, so an individual born with just one kidney can still live a normal life.

The kidneys work as filters, retaining materials the body needs from the blood and putting them back in the body's circulation. Wastes and harmful products like toxins are passed out as urine and excreted by the body. The kidneys also monitor the body's need for water and *electrolytes,* such as sodium, potassium, chloride, and bicarbonate. Electrolytes help keep the body's systems balanced. By saving or excreting electrolytes and other materials as needed, the kidneys play a valuable role in maintaining a constant healthy environment for the body.

The main functioning unit of the kidney is the *nephron* which acts as a filtering system for the body. Each kidney is made up of about 1 million nephrons, each consisting of a group of blood vessels formed into a cuplike structure, the glomerulus. The glomerulus is attached to a structure called a tubule; together, one glomerulus and one tubule form one nephron.

Blood is filtered in the capillaries (tiny arteries) of the glomerulus, and red blood cells and proteins are retained. The fluid that remains passes through the tubule, where sodium, potassium, and water are secreted or reabsorbed, depending on the body's needs. This small tubule joins with other tubules, which lead to larger and larger tubules. Eventually, the large tubules empty into the ureter.

The amount of fluid taken in or lost (through vomiting or diarrhea, for example), type of diet, any medications taken, and exposure to extreme temperatures all affect the amount and type of urine produced. The urine is then transported to the urinary bladder through the ureters. The bladder is a sac of muscle located in the middle of the lower abdomen behind the pubic bone. The bladder's main function is to act as a storage bin for urine. The amount the bladder can hold varies from person to person. Once the bladder has reached its capacity, the urine passes into the urethra, a tube which is 2 to 3 inches long in women. Then, it exits the body from a small opening above the vagina.

Urination is a two-step process: First, the walls of your bladder begin to stretch because it is full. This stretching sends signals to the brain that it is time to urinate. Second, when you are ready to urinate, you relax the urinary sphincter muscle at the base of the bladder around the urethra. This allows urine to pass. The amount of urine varies anywhere from less than an ounce to a cup or more.

The muscles that provide support for the pelvic organs (the bladder, uterus, and rectum) also assist the workings of the urinary tract. Although they are a part of the musculoskeletal system, they are important in maintaining bladder control. If these muscles weaken and sag, incontinence, or loss of urinary control, can result.

In women, the urinary and reproductive pathways are separate. In men, the urethra transports not only urine but also semen. The urethra in women is shorter than that in men, which means women are more likely to have some urinary problems, such as infections.

KEEPING THE URINARY SYSTEM HEALTHY

To keep your urinary system healthy, drink plenty of water. Water plays many important roles in the healthy functioning of your urinary tract. The amount of water in your body helps the urinary system determine whether more electrolytes, such as sodium, should be retained or excreted. When the concentration of electrolytes is too high, your body releases a hormone that causes water retention and stimulates your feelings of thirst. The kidney then gets rid of the excess electrolytes and water.

Drinking enough water allows you to produce a large quantity of urine. You should drink enough fluids,

Figure 2.1 The Urinary System
The urinary system is composed of the *kidneys*, two fist-sized organs on either side of the body; the *ureters*, tubes that lead from the kidneys to the *bladder*, where urine is stored; and the *urethra*, through which urine is passed to the outside of the body. The kidneys play a vital role in filtering waste products and maintaining chemical and electrical balances within the body. Each kidney is covered with an outer *capsule* made up of strong fibrous tissue. Inside the capsule, the *cortex* and the *medulla* contain specialized structures that collect and process fluids, waste, and metabolic products. Blood is supplied from the *renal artery*, which branches off from the central *abdominal aorta*, and drained by the *renal vein*, which joins the *vena cava* before returning to the heart.

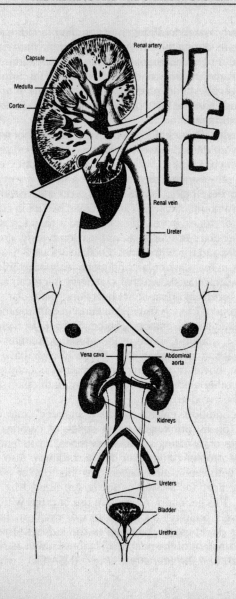

particularly water, to allow emptying the bladder every 3 to 4 hours during the day. At least half of the fluid each day should be noncarbonated water. (Carbonation can worsen some urinary conditions.) Although the urinary tract is usually sterile, producing large amounts of urine helps wash harmful bacteria out of the urinary system if they should enter.

Usually, if your kidneys work well, you do not need to limit your diet. If, however, you have high blood pressure—which is linked with some kinds of kidney disease—a salt-restricted diet may be prescribed. If you are prone to developing kidney stones, you may need to limit the amount of calcium and oxalate, two main components of stones, in your diet. Calcium is found in milk and other diary products, as well as some leafy, green vegetables and fish with bones. Oxalate is found in large amounts in tea, dark colas, and green leafy vegetables.

Research has shown that cranberry juice can help prevent recurrent urinary tract infections, particularly in older women. There is usually no harm in drinking moderate quantities of cranberry juice. Since it is a good source of vitamin C—one of the essential vitamins—it can be a part of a good diet. If you already have an infection, however, drinking large amounts of cranberry juice or other acidic juices may aggravate the pain and should be avoided.

A condition called "irritable bladder" may be brought on by drinking a lot of coffee or carbonated beverages or by eating acidic, spicy foods. If you tend to have this problem, alter your diet accordingly. Also, be careful with medications, even over-the-counter products. Medications as well as toxins are filtered by the kidneys. This generally allows safe use of drugs without high levels building up in the blood. Even so, large amounts of drugs can build up in the kidneys. This is particularly true of the pain medications known as *nonsteroidal anti-inflammatory drugs* (NSAIDs), which include ibuprofen and naproxen. If you take these drugs for a long time, you may damage your kidneys.

Good hygiene is also helpful. Because a woman's urethra is very close to the vagina and fairly close to the rectum, infections can be passed from one of these openings to the others. Wiping from the front to back after defecating helps prevent infecting the urethra with bacteria that are normally present in the vagina or rectum. For the same reason, women who are prone to infections should avoid tub baths and douches.

Good hygiene after intercourse is also important. During intercourse, bacteria from the vagina or from the man's penis can enter the urethra. Cleansing the genital area after having sex helps prevent this. Urinating after intercourse helps to flush bacteria out of the bladder and urethra before they can build up and cause an infection. This is most helpful when the quantity of urine is large enough to create a good stream to wash out the bladder.

Smoking tobacco increases the risk of some urinary tract conditions. Tobacco smoking is also associated with atherosclerosis, including the blood vessels, that go to the kidney. This can cause high blood pressure and loss of kidney function. Smoking tends to cause chronic coughing, which can add to problems with bladder control. It also increases the risk of bladder cancer—which can occur even years after a woman has quit smoking. The best thing is not to start smoking in the first place. If you do smoke, quit.

COMMON URINARY PROBLEMS

Problems affecting the urinary system are common. Certain symptoms are related to specific problems. Recognizing symptoms can help you decide whether or not you need to see a doctor. Your regular doctor can treat some problems, but others may require referral to a specialist (see "Who Treats the Urinary System?").

Some urinary tract symptoms affect just the urine. For example, the urine may be bloody or unusually colored, or you may feel you need to urinate right away (urgency) or more often than usual (frequency). In other cases, urination is painful. Some symptoms affect other

WHO TREATS THE URINARY SYSTEM?

If you have such urinary symptoms as pain, bloody urine, or frequent urination, you can be treated by any one of several kinds of doctors. An internist or a family physician can diagnose and treat simple problems, such as infections, and refer you to a nephrologist or a urologist for more specialized care if needed.

A *nephrologist* is a medical doctor who specializes in problems affecting the kidney. She or he is a specialist in internal medicine with advanced training in kidney disease, unbalanced electrolytes, kidney failure, and other problems connected to the kidneys, such as high blood pressure or swelling. A *urologist* is a surgeon who specializes in the structure of the urinary system, the drainage of the kidneys, and the function of the bladder. If the kidneys fail, nephrologists and urologists both can be involved with diagnosis and treatment. If artificially filtering the blood (dialysis) is needed, a nephrologist supervises the whole process.

Some urinary problems, such as infection and bladder control, can be treated by your gynecologist as well.

parts of the body: high blood pressure, fever and chills, back pain, or puffy hands, feet, or eyes. Some women have no symptoms at all, even if a kidney is slowly beginning to fail. When this happens, the body has adjusted to the failing kidney and so there are no symptoms. Other women may have severe symptoms caused by relatively minor problems that are easily treated. The severity of the symptoms is not always a good indication of the seriousness of disease.

Symptoms

Bloody Urine

Normal urine is pale to medium yellow. Blood in the urine (hematuria) is a sign that a serious condition may be present. It should prompt you to see a doctor as soon as possible. The urine may be bright red with clots, a light pink, gray, or dark brown like tea or cola. The color depends on the amount of blood, how "old" the urine is, and how acidic. Even if the urine is not an unusual color, small amounts of blood can be present. Although invisible to the naked eye, the blood can be seen if the urine is examined with special paper (dipstick) or under a microscope.

An infection of the urinary tract is the most common cause of hematuria. Fever and urinary pain, frequency and urgency of urination also are common with infection. Other causes of bloody urine include trauma and injury, kidney diseases, such as glomerulonephritis, stones, and tumors (mostly cancers). Blood in the urine also can be caused by very strenuous exercise, such as jogging (particularly very long distances). It is important to have a further evaluation to determine the cause. In some cases, no cause can be found.

Because a woman's urethra is close to her vagina and rectum, bloody urine can sometimes reflect blood from these structures rather than blood from the urinary system. Finally, the red or brown colored urine may be caused by medication, some forms of liver disease, or even, in some people, a recent serving of beets.

Pain

One frequent cause of pain is a urinary tract infection. When a kidney is infected, the pain is felt in the upper back or side, and fever and chills may occur. If the pain is low and in front and occurs mostly when you are urinating, it is more likely to be a bladder infection.

Another bladder condition, called interstitial cystitis, can cause pain. If you have pain when you urinate and chronic pain in the genital area (for example, the clitoris, the labia, and the vagina) or the thighs or lower back, you may be suffering from this condition.

Stones in the urinary tract are another cause of pain. Such pain is spasmodic and can travel from the back down the side into the vaginal lips. Although stones in the kidneys do not usually cause pain, when stones leave the kidneys and pass down the ureter, they can cause severe pain that has been described as worse than labor pains. This is called renal colic.

Urinary Urgency and Frequency

A strong feeling that you must urinate is called urinary urgency. Urinary frequency is the need to void often. Both are common symptoms of a urinary tract infection or interstitial cystitis. Urgency and frequency are not always linked to disease, however. In cold weather it is common for people to void often. Pregnant women typically experience an increased need to urinate as the uterus grows, causing pressure on the bladder.

COMMON CONDITIONS AFFECTING THE URINARY TRACT

Some urinary tract conditions are minor problems that can be easily treated. Others can seriously harm the body's ability to function and can even be life-threatening if they are not caught in time.

Urinary system conditions can be grouped into the following types:

- Infections
- Irritations or inflammations
- Stones
- Urinary incontinence
- Kidney failure
- Nephrotic syndrome
- Inherited kidney disease
- Tumors
- Systemic disorders

INFECTIONS

Bacteria are normally present in some parts of the body, such as the vagina and rectum, but not in the urine. When bacteria invade a part of the urinary system, infections can occur. Women are more likely to have urinary tract infections than men, because a woman's urethra, vagina, and rectum are all close together and her urethra is fairly short. It is relatively easy for bacteria from the vagina or rectum to travel up the urethra into the bladder and then to the kidneys.

Since common symptoms of frequency and painful urination can occur with other urinary conditions, a diagnosis of infection cannot be made on the basis of symptoms alone. Diagnosis depends on examination of a urine specimen and obtaining a urine culture. If pus cells are seen in the urine and bacteria can be grown in the urine culture, then infection is likely the cause.

Usually, infections that are not complicated by other problems can be easily treated with antibiotics. The antibiotic needed for treatment can be determined by studying the urine culture. When medicine is prescribed, take all the pills, even if symptoms disappear before all the medication has been taken. Stopping antibiotics too soon increases the chance that the infection will recur.

Bladder Infection

Cystitis or bladder infection is the most common urinary tract infection. Because of the proximity of the vagina and the urethra, it is not unusual for bladder infections to begin when a woman becomes sexually active. Some women are particularly prone to these infections. They may have more aggressive bacteria, or they may lack needed defense mechanisms to fight off the infection.

Sexual intercourse itself may prompt a bladder infection. Sometimes you can have symptoms within hours of having sex, sometimes days later. The typical symptoms of a bladder infection are frequency, urgency, and pain with urination. The urine may be bloody or cloudy, or it may have an unusual odor.

A bladder infection is diagnosed by examining a urine sample and obtaining a urine culture. Most bladder infections not associated with a kidney infection can be cured within 3 to 5 days by using antibiotics. You can help the process by increasing the amount of water you drink and urinating often.

Kidney Infection

Kidney infections often start with bacteria in the bladder. The bacteria travel up the ureters to the kidney and cause the infection. When kidney infections recur, the cause may be reflux, the backing up of urine from the bladder to the kidneys. This is caused by a faulty valve mechanism where the bladder and the ureter join. Other causes of recurrent kidney infections are stones, diabetes mellitus, and previous scarring.

Kidney infection is also called *pyelonephritis* and is much less common than bladder infection. If you have a kidney infection, you may first experience urinary urgency and frequency. Later symptoms are fever and chills, pain in the upper back or side, nausea, and sometimes vomiting.

Diagnosis

A clean catch urine specimen and urine culture are examined to make the diagnosis. An X-ray or ultrasound of the kidney can help determine if an obstruction exists that could make the infection more serious. Also, a special X-ray of the bladder can identify infections caused by reflux.

Treatment

Sometimes, a kidney infection disappears spontaneously. However, because complications may occur if it doesn't, all kidney infections should be treated by a physician with antibiotics. Drinking large amounts of water, although helpful for other reasons, cannot flush infection out of the kidney. Antibiotics should be taken for 7–14 days to prevent complications. If you are too ill to take pills or if the infection is severe, you will be treated in the hospital with intravenous medication.

Hospital treatment is usually required if a woman has both a serious kidney infection and a urinary obstruction caused, for example, by stones. While most kidney infections heal with proper treatment, complications such as shock, bloodstream infection, and abscess formation may occur. The kidneys may become scarred and may fail to function properly. When stones or other obstructions occur along with infection, both intravenous antibiotics and relief of the blockage by surgery are needed.

IRRITATIONS AND INFLAMMATIONS

Bladder infections are only one type of cystitis. The symptoms of urinary frequency, urgency, and painful urination can also be caused by other types of cystitis, including irritation, or inflammation, of the bladder. These conditions are not caused by bacterial infection.

Irritable Bladder

Irritable bladder refers to an irritation of the lining of the bladder that is not caused by bacteria. It is also known as cystitis, chronic urethritis, trigonitis, or urethral syndrome.

Certain foods and beverages can cause the symptoms of irritable bladder; for example, too much coffee, carbonated beverages, or foods and beverages that are acidic or spicy. Some women also find their symptoms made worse by sex, emotional stress, and changes in their hormones that occur just before their menstrual periods. When irritable bladder is suspected, you should have a pelvic exam in addition to the usual urine studies.

For doctors and patients alike, irritable bladder can be a frustrating condition. The symptoms are similar to those of a bacterial infection. It is not unusual for symptoms to improve while you are taking antibiotics and then become worse when you stop. Antibiotics may seem to improve the condition because they are usually taken with extra water. When the course of antibiotics is completed, most people return to their normal drinking habits—often not enough water—and symptoms return. Antibiotics, however, do not usually provide a lasting cure and can be harmful. Taking antibiotics for weeks to months can lead to the development of recurrent yeast infections in the vagina.

More water intake is the best treatment. Increase your water intake whenever you begin to have symptoms of bladder irritability. Self-treatment begins with drinking 8 ounces of water every 20–30 minutes for 2–3 hours. This usually promotes a good washout of bacteria or other irritants. You may also find it helpful to keep a diary indicating when symptoms occur and what seems to cause them. Once the cause has been identified, often it can be avoided. Warm baths to relax the pelvic muscles may be soothing, too.

If increased water intake does not eliminate the symptoms, pills can be prescribed (phenazopyridine hydrochloride) that make the inside of the bladder numb. This medication changes the color of the urine to orange. Physical therapy may also help.

Interstitial Cystitis

Women who have interstitial cystitis have not only urinary frequency, urgency, and pain with urination but also chronic pelvic pain. When symptoms are severe, you may urinate every 10–15 minutes, day and night, trying to eliminate the pain and the intense need to urinate. The intense pain is often temporarily relieved by urination. Because of the pain, this condition is also referred to as painful bladder syndrome.

The cause of interstitial cystitis is not known, but it occurs more often in women than in men. Like irritable bladder, stress and changes in hormone levels both seem to initiate the symptoms.

Diagnosis

The diagnosis of interstitial cystitis begins with a taking of your medical history. You may have a history of recurrent bladder infections. The evaluation includes urine studies and a pelvic exam. When a cystoscopy (a look inside the bladder with a special instrument) is done, its findings are usually normal. Your symptoms and the negative cystoscopy confirm the diagnosis.

Treatment

The symptoms can be minimized or controlled by a variety of treatments. Options include the increased water intake described for irritable bladder. For some women, medications may be effective, including:

- Phenazopyridine hydrochloride
- Tricyclic antidepressants (amitriptyline, doxepin, nortriptyline)
- Antihistamines
- Calcium channel blockers

Placing medications directly in the bladder helps more than half of women with this condition. Medications used this way include:

- Dimethyl sulfoxide
- Steroids
- Heparin

Because changes in hormone levels seem to provoke symptoms, medications that change hormone levels— such as birth control pills—can be an important part of treatment. After you go through menopause, you stop producing the female hormone estrogen. Replacing this hormone with medication is generally helpful. Counseling or biofeedback therapy to improve stress management can help, too.

STONES

Stones are composed of substances normally found in the urine (for example, calcium, oxalate, and uric acid) which have built up in high concentration. Although they are produced in the kidneys, stones can be found anywhere in the urinary tract. Stones in the kidneys usually do not cause symptoms, however. Stones are more commonly found in the bladder or the ureter, where they can cause great pain.

Stones in the urinary tract can be present for a long time and not cause pain until they obstruct excretion. A stone in the ureter can prevent the passage of urine. When this happens, urine continues to be produced and the part of the urinary tract above the stone dilates (expands) with the urine that cannot escape. This expansion of the urinary tract causes severe pain, which may radiate into the groin and vulva. Nausea, vomiting, and fever can occur as well. (See Fig. 2.2)

Pain from kidney stones is worse when they are being passed; therefore, the pain seems to come and go intermittently. The stone temporarily blocks off the ureter, causing pain, then moves slightly, allowing urine to pass. This gives temporary relief until the stone lodges again in a position that blocks the ureter.

The type and location of the stone may be linked to the cause. Some stones are commonly associated with infection and certain bacteria. The tendency to form certain types of stones may be inherited, as in the case of the uric acid stones and cysteine stones. Still other stones are formed as a result of another medical condition, such as calcium stones in patients with overactive parathyroid glands, or as a complication of leukemia or chemotherapy for lymphoma.

Risk factors for stone formation are dehydration (not drinking enough water), excessive sweating, excessive calcium intake, and prolonged bed rest. Individuals who have had a severe injury and need long periods of bed rest are prone to having stones. For unknown reasons, men are more likely to form stones than women.

Diagnosis

Stones can be suspected on the basis of intermittent sharp, knifelike pains. To diagnose stones, doctors use X-rays of the urinary tract or methods that allow them to view the urinary tract directly. Stone composition can be determined by analysis of the urine and the stone.

Treatment

Most stones eventually pass into the bladder and require no treatment except pain medication. Stones smaller than one-quarter inch usually pass on their own; stones larger than one-half inch often require treatment. Treatment may include methods to dissolve or remove

Figure 2.2 Kidney Stones and Polyps
Stones in the urinary tract can result from infections or disorders that cause excessive excretion of certain types of waste products that may begin to crystallize and form granules and eventually larger stones. Stones in the ureter can cause a great deal of pain as the ureter contracts in an attempt to pass them. Polyps are usually benign masses of tissue that form inside the bladder.

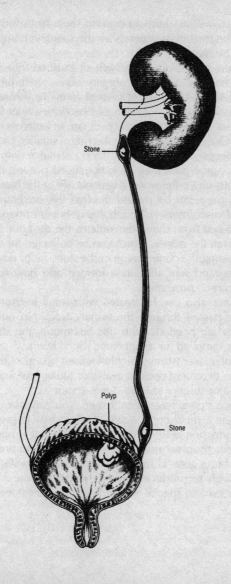

stones as well as drugs to prevent them from forming again. The treatment depends on the size and composition of the stone.

Often stones can be broken or crushed into sand inside the body without surgery. This procedure is referred to as lithotripsy. Different forms of lithotripsy are available, many of which can be done under local anesthesia in a doctor's office or an ambulatory care center. Once the stone is broken into smaller pieces, these pieces pass without further assistance into the bladder. Some pain may be experienced passing these fragments. Once the stone fragments are in the bladder, though, they can be passed through the urethra with minimal discomfort. After lithotripsy is performed, the urine passed from the body contains the dust and fragments from the stones, which can be collected for studies. Knowing the composition of the stone helps doctors to understand why the stone formed and how future stones can be prevented.

Stones also can be treated with small instruments that are passed through the urinary tract. No outside incisions are needed. With this technique, the stones can be removed or fragmented by lithotripsy or by means of a laser (strong, highly focused beams of light). With the treatment options available today, few women need major surgery to have stones removed.

Once stones have been treated, you can take steps to prevent a recurrence. Again, the best way to prevent stone formation is to drink plenty of water. It is hard to know exactly how much you need to drink to prevent stones, but a general rule is to drink enough water and other fluids to produce about 2 quarts of urine a day. Medication and special diet can help prevent stones.

URINARY INCONTINENCE

Urinary incontinence is the involuntary excretion of urine. The amount of urine may be as little as a few drops or as much as the entire contents of the bladder. Although urinary incontinence can happen at any age, it is more likely in women after they have had children and after menopause.

Our aging population means that incontinence is a concern for many women today. Adult diaper and other types of pads are a growing business. These products help prevent embarrassment from leaks, but they do not cure the problem. Many ways to improve or cure bladder problems exist, however. Most women can free themselves from relying on pads with appropriate treatment.

To maintain control of your bladder, a balance must be struck between the bladder and the bladder outlet. The bladder outlet consists of the urethra plus the pelvic muscles that surround the urethra. These muscles are also called the pelvic floor muscles. When the bladder contracts, it allows the urine to empty. When the bladder outlet contracts, it prevents urine from passing. To prevent urine from leaking, the bladder outlet keeps up a high pressure as the bladder is filling and at times of stress (for example, coughing, lifting, or bending). Any time the bladder's contractions exceed those of the bladder outlet, urine leaks.

There are several types of urinary incontinence:

- *Stress* incontinence is urine loss that occurs when the bladder outlet's pressure is exceeded. Coughing, sneezing, bending, and lifting are some actions that can cause this form of incontinence.

- *Urge* incontinence is linked with having a strong urge to urinate and being unable to get to the toilet in time.

- *Spontaneous* incontinence involves urine loss for no identifiable reason. There is no sense of urgency or specific activity linked to the leakage.

- *Enuresis, or bedwetting,* is common in children, but it tends to resolve with age. When enuresis occurs in an adult, there is generally some neurological problem causing the loss of bladder control.

The common causes of urinary incontinence are weak pelvic floor muscles, an overactive bladder muscle, inability to completely empty the bladder, and neurological diseases such as strokes, multiple sclerosis, or Parkinson's disease. In older women, restricted mobility, low levels of estrogen after menopause, inability to recognize that the bladder is full, and multiple medications are important causes. (See Fig. 2.3)

Diagnosis

The diagnosis of incontinence begins with the taking of your medical history. You may be asked to complete a diary that shows when you drank fluids, when you urinated, whether urine was leaked (and if so, how much), and what you were doing when the urine leaked. A urine sample is examined for blood or signs of infection. When blood is found, a kidney X-ray and cystoscopy are needed to rule out other problems.

A pelvic exam is done to allow the doctor to look for signs in the tissues that too little estrogen is being produced. (Lack of estrogen can weaken the pelvic floor muscles.) The doctor can also check the pelvic floor muscles and determine whether they are providing enough support to the base of the bladder and the urethra. Weakness in the pelvic floor muscles can allow the bladder and urethra to sag into the vaginal space. Sagging of just the bladder is called a cystocele, while sagging of both the bladder and the urethra is called a cystourethrocele.

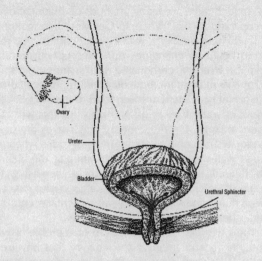

Figure 2.3 Incontinence
One cause of urinary incontinence in older women is decreased production of estrogen at menopause. This decrease can cause the muscular wall of the bladder to thicken, which makes it able to hold less urine and can cause leakage of urine.

Even if blood is not found in the urine, cystoscopy may be done to look at the lining of the bladder and to examine the position and function of the urethra. Often, special studies of bladder function called urodynamics are done to check bladder sensation, bladder capacity, presence of abnormal bladder contractions, and ability of the bladder to empty.

Treatment
The first step in treating urinary incontinence is to see a physician. Many women suffer with this problem needlessly because they are either embarrassed or do not want to have surgery, which they think is the only

cure. In fact, there are many methods of treatment other than operations (see "Where to Get More Information").

If you have problems with bladder control, you may wish to begin by changing your diet. As with irritable bladder, coffee, tea, carbonated drinks, and acidic spicy food and drinks can increase bladder irritability and add to incontinence. Many women tend to cut back on the amount of water they drink, thinking that this will help prevent leakage. On the contrary, this makes the problem worse. The concentrated urine that forms when not enough water is drunk is more irritating to the bladder than diluted urine. Therefore, slowly increasing the amount of water drunk each day is a good idea. You can expect that urinary frequency may increase until the bladder becomes used to the extra water.

You can make other changes to ease problems with incontinence and improve the chance that any treatment will succeed. Chronic coughing and constipation strain the system and should be avoided. Also, try to become aware of any habits you have in sports or at work that can affect the delicate balance of bladder control. For example, don't strain to lift heavy weights.

Bladder training is also important. In bladder training, you go to the bathroom on a regular schedule whether or not you feel the need to urinate. You start off with a schedule of urinating every hour, and gradually increase the intervals between urinating.

Doing special exercises can help you strengthen your pelvic floor muscles. These exercises, sometimes called Kegel exercises, require you to identify and squeeze a certain group of muscles. A doctor or nurse can explain how the exercises are to be done and check that they are being performed correctly. A positive effect is usually seen after 6 weeks of performing 10–20 10-second contractions 4 times a day. (You may only be able to hold the contractions 2–3 seconds at first but can gradually work up to 10 seconds.) Biofeedback can also help with pelvic muscle exercises. A small device is placed in the vagina to measure the contractions of the muscles and give you immediate feedback when you are squeezing the right muscle.

Small weights, called vaginal cones, can be used with the exercises. They help you learn which muscles to contract and can increase the strength of the pelvic floor muscles. You insert a weight into your vagina and then use your pelvic muscles to prevent it from falling out. Hold the weight in for 15 minutes at a time and do the exercise twice a day. These weights are available without a prescription, but they work best after you have learned how to use them properly from a doctor or nurse.

If you have problems with bladder control because your pelvic organs sag, it can be helpful to use a contraceptive diaphragm when you are doing a physically stressful activity like jogging or playing volleyball or tennis. The diaphragm helps give the urethra the support the pelvic muscles lack. The use of the diaphragm should be combined with pelvic muscle exercises to strengthen the muscles.

The newest form of treatment is electrical stimulation of the pelvic muscles. Although its use is fairly common in Europe, it is just becoming available in the United States.

Medications can also improve urinary control. Some drugs relax the bladder muscle, allowing it to store large volumes of urine and prevent uncontrollable bladder contractions. Common examples are oxybutynin chloride, propantheline, hyoscyamine, and imipramine. If you take these medications, be alert for constipation, a side effect that can make urinary incontinence worse. Other medications work by increasing the strength of the bladder outlet. This type is commonly found in over-the-counter cold medications whose active ingredients are pseudoephedrine and phenylpropanolamine.

Estrogen replacement therapy may also help. Estrogen helps the bladder and urethra to function normally and improves the strength of the pelvic muscles. Estrogen creams placed in the vagina probably provide the most immediate improvement in the urinary tract, but pills and patches are available, too. Use the medications along with a bladder training program and pelvic muscle exercises.

When bladder training, exercises, and medications are not successful, surgery is usually needed. Surgery can be performed regardless of age. The goal of surgery is to lift the bladder and urethra back to their normal position and prevent them from sagging into the vagina. The surgery does not strengthen the pelvic floor muscles, however.

Many types of surgery may be done, and the selection depends on the surgeon's experience and preference as well as factors individual to the woman. In general, 50–60 percent of women remain dry, with good bladder control, 5 years after the operation.

A new option is injection of material around the urethra to support it. A relatively minor operation compared to some other types of surgical treatment, it can be done with local anesthesia.

After treatment, try to adopt healthy habits that do not strain the muscles and bladder:

- Quit smoking.
- Get treatment for chronic respiratory conditions.
- Avoid heavy lifting when possible.
- Avoid becoming constipated.

You can prevent having urinary incontinence if you perform routine pelvic muscle exercises throughout your life. Once learned, these exercises can easily be made a part of your daily routine. They can be performed while driving, waiting in line at the grocery store, or brushing your teeth. Taking estrogen at menopause, if recommended by a doctor, can also help prevent incontinence.

KIDNEY FAILURE (RENAL FAILURE)

Acute Kidney Failure
(Acute Renal Failure)

In acute renal failure the kidneys stop functioning suddenly. This almost never occurs in otherwise healthy women. The most common causes are shock due to infection, bleeding, severe dehydration, exposure to toxins, drugs, or abnormalities in the arteries in the kidneys. Acute renal failure can occur in pregnant women who have severe high blood pressure.

In some cases, acute kidney failure can be reversed if the correct diagnosis is made and the right therapy is promptly started. In other cases, kidney failure lasts for about 10 days before recovery begins. Rarely, women do not recover and develop end-stage kidney disease.

Kidney failure is usually part of a long, continuous process. The initial damage may be slight but progress until all the nephrons are damaged. Or, healthy nephrons may work harder to compensate for the damaged nephrons, and after years they become damaged from overwork. This leads to further decline in function, so a vicious cycle is established, leading to chronic renal failure.

Chronic Kidney Failure
(Chronic Renal Failure)

The rate at which kidney function declines varies from person to person. In conditions like polycystic kidney disease or diabetes the process is protracted over decades. Rapid kidney failure, of months to a few years, occurs in HIV-associated kidney disease and some patients with lupus.

Women with failing kidneys usually show no symptoms until the failure is well advanced. The only signs may be high blood pressure or abnormal laboratory results if blood and urine are examined. Once the kidneys are working at only 15–20 percent of normal capacity, however, most women begin to develop symptoms. As the kidneys continue to fail, symptoms worsen and can include fatigue, increasing shortness of breath, nausea, vomiting, diarrhea, problems thinking clearly, poor memory, muscle weakness, abnormal muscle twitching, anemia, easy bruising, itching, and bleeding from the gums, stomach, and intestines. There may also be dehydration or swelling. Menstruation can become irregular and eventually stop. Sex drive diminishes. Although conception can take place, pregnancy in patients with chronic kidney disease is very risky for the mother. Live births occur in women with renal transplants, but rarely in women treated with dialysis. Without treatment, such as dialysis or transplant, women with severe symptoms eventually develop seizures, coma, and death.

Today, there are effective treatments for kidney failure, all of which require professional care with a nephrologist. If your kidneys are not functioning well, your daily fluid intake may be limited so you don't drink more fluids than your kidneys can process, and you may be asked to weigh yourself daily. Amounts of sodium and potassium in the diet are often restricted for the same reasons. If too much protein is eaten, the symptoms of uremia are worsened. The nephrologist will recommend a renal dietician to work with you to plan a diet.

Recent research suggests that early in kidney failure, medication (angiotensin-converting enzyme [ACE] (inhibitors) can prevent the development of kidney failure or end-stage renal disease (ESRD). The main treatments for ESRD are dialysis and transplantation (see "Dialysis—The Artificial Kidney").

End-Stage Renal Disease (ESRD)

End-stage kidney disease occurs when kidney function is so poor that a person cannot survive without aggressive treatment. The severe symptoms are known as uremia and include

- Malaise
- Fatigue and disturbed sleep
- Nausea, vomiting, and diarrhea
- Loss of appetite and sex drive
- Inability to concentrate
- Itching
- Swelling
- Shortness of breath

In more advanced cases (rarely seen today, due to early treatment), uremia causes twitching, muscle jerks, increased skin color, chest pains, seizures, bleeding and bruising, or coma. Patients with uremia appear wasted (overly thin), and their skin may be pale or yellow. Their breath smells like wine, with a distinctively bad odor. In advanced cases, the skin may be covered with a white frost, and the person may exhibit a flapping tremor when the hands are raised. Fortunately, aggressive, early treatment with dialysis or a transplant can prevent these types of severe symptoms.

Dialysis—The Artificial Kidney

In dialysis, filtering that is normally done by the kidneys is done by an artificial method. There are two types: hemodialysis and peritoneal dialysis. Dialysis is started when serious or uncomfortable symptoms cannot be managed by more conservative methods. It is a chronic form of treatment. Once it is begun, it must be continued to prevent uremia. The effectiveness of dialysis usually depends on your general health and your willingness to cooperate with this chronic therapy. If you receive a kidney transplant, dialysis is no longer needed.

Hemodialysis

If hemodialysis is selected, a minor operation is performed to create permanent access to the blood system. Blood can then be pumped into the dialysis machine for filtering and purification and then back to the patient. Treatments usually last 4–5 hours and are needed three times a week, but this depends on your size and other factors. Although you can be taught to perform dialysis at home, most people go to dialysis centers for treatment. (See Fig. 2.4)

The chronic and time-consuming nature of dialysis requires careful planning and scheduling and often requires you to make changes in your life. It may interfere with working unless your schedule is very flexible. It is necessary, for example, to plan in advance for trips away from home. Usually a temporary referral to another dialysis center can be arranged.

Peritoneal Dialysis

Peritoneal dialysis, sometimes called continuous ambulatory peritoneal dialysis (CAPD), also requires a point

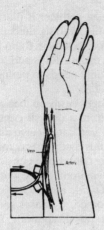

Figure 2.4 Dialysis

Dialysis allows the filtering of bodily fluids that is normally done by the kidneys to be done artificially (below). In hemodialysis, blood is pumped from an artery through a machine, where it is cleansed and then returned to the body through a vein (left). Waste products are filtered out of the blood through a membrane, while substances needed by the body remain in the blood.

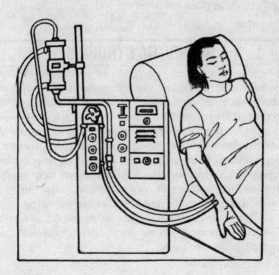

of access to the body. In this case, a catheter is placed surgically in the abdomen so sterile dialysis fluid can flow in and out. The fluid is allowed to remain there for 6–8 hours. When it is drained out, excess fluids and toxins are drained out with it. The patient needs to perform 4 such exchanges a day. (See Fig. 2.5)

This type of dialysis can be taught easily so that you can do it at home. If you live far from a dialysis center, this may be the only practical way you can receive dialysis. Because infection is a risk of this method, you must carefully follow the procedures described by your doctor. As long as you are in a clean environment, you can perform this technique at home, at work, or on vacation.

While the fluid is in the abdomen, it causes some slight abdominal distension but no discomfort. The swelling is not noticeable, and the presence of the catheter tube does not interfere with sexual activity.

NEPHROTIC SYNDROME

In nephrotic syndrome, serum proteins pass into the urine because of damage to the glomerulus of the nephron. This condition, formerly known as nephrosis, is associated with swelling and abnormal laboratory test results. Along with treatment for the specific causes of nephrotic syndrome, alterations in diet can help in managing this condition. Low salt intake can help control the swelling, and the amount of protein in the diet must be increased to make up for that lost in the urine.

The most common causes of nephrotic syndrome are various forms of glomerulonephritis, diabetes, lupus, and multiple myeloma.

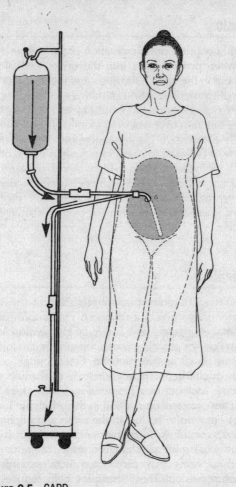

Figure 2.5 CAPD
Continuous ambulatory peritoneal dialysis (CAPD) allows the filtering of excess fluid and waste when this function cannot be done efficiently by the kidneys. Dialysis fluid flows in and out of the abdomen through a catheter that is placed surgically. The fluid must be replaced every 6-8 hours.

Diagnosis

Glomerulonephritis, or inflammation of the glomerulus, occurs when protein leaks into the urine. Red blood cells appear in the urine. Diagnosis and identification of the type of glomerulonephritis requires a kidney biopsy. In some cases, glomerulonephritis causes rapid decline in kidney function over weeks to months. This is known as rapidly progressive glomerulonephritis. Uncommon but severe, it is linked to conditions such as AIDS, other forms of glomerulonephritis, high blood pressure in pregnancy, and lupus. A kidney biopsy is nearly always needed to make a quick, accurate diagnosis. Prompt treatment is needed to prevent irreversible damage to the kidneys.

Treatment

Common types of glomerulonephritis are post-streptoccal glomerulonephritis, membranous glomerulonephritis, minimal change disease, and focal glomerulosclerosis (FGS). Post-streptoccal glomerulonephritis can follow a strep sore throat or skin infection. Once thought to be a disease of children, it is now diagnosed in adults and the elderly. Membranous glomerulonephritis does not usually cause microscopic blood in the urine, but it can still cause protein to be lost in the urine and nephrotic syndrome to occur. A kidney biopsy can distinguish this condition from minimal change disease. Membranous glomerulonephritis may be treated with steroids or immunosuppression. These therapies help reduce the amount of protein passed in the urine and prevent kidney failure from occurring. However, up to 40 percent of people with this condition improve even without treatment. If no other cause is found, membranous glomerulonephritis may be linked with cancer, such as lung cancer or cancer of the stomach or intestines. Focal glomerulonephritis is one of the most common causes of glomerulonephritis, and it is increasing in frequency. It responds poorly to treatment with immunosuppression, and renal failure generally occurs after some years. FGS behaves differently in patients with HIV, being associated with rapidly developing renal failure.

Those who have swelling, abnormal amounts of protein in their urine, and nephrotic syndrome have minimal change disease if a standard kidney biopsy appears to be normal. When the same kidney tissue sampled is examined under an electron microscope, changes are seen. This condition also can be treated with steroids or immunosuppressants. While it sometimes disappears without treatment, it may recur even after successful therapy. Although repeated treatment may be needed, it rarely leads to kidney failure. Sometimes, minimal change disease is linked to lymphomas.

TRANSPLANTATION—THE GIFT OF LIFE

The successful transplantation of a kidney restores normal function. With a transplant, a woman does not need dialysis or any restrictions to the diet.

Special tests are done prior to a transplantation to match the patient with the kidney least likely to be rejected. Blood from the donor and the patient is tested for tissue type, the presence of antibodies, and other factors that affect the likelihood of rejection.

The best match is a kidney donated by an identical twin. Women who are identical twins share the same immune systems, which makes them likely to accept each other's organs. A kidney from another family member may succeed as well, especially if both the donor and the recipient have the same tissue types. Blood-related (true) brothers or sisters are the best match after an identical twin, followed by parents or children. A living kidney donor must have two normal kidneys (since only one healthy kidney is needed by the body) and be in good health, with no signs of disease, psychological problems, or infection. If no match is available in the family, a kidney from an unrelated, deceased donor (cadaver donor) can be used. Cadaver donation is the most common form.

The body's immune system responds to a transplanted organ as it would to any foreign material. It would destroy the new kidney if there were not some way to suppress the immune system. To do this, medications must be taken that suppress the immune system enough to prevent rejection of the organ, but not completely. Complete suppression of the immune system would leave the person open to disease. Those taking immunosuppressive drugs are more likely to have problems with infection since the immune system is less able to fight off the invader.

Your nephrologist will help you select a transplant center. The center should do at least 40 kidney transplants each year. The United Network of Organ Sharing (see "Where to Get More Information") can help provide assistance.

Some people are not candidates for a transplant. They include those who:

- Are unable to tolerate the operation
- Have an infection that cannot be treated
- Are infected with HIV or have AIDS
- Are likely to have recurrent kidney disease in the transplanted kidney
- Are unable to take the needed immunosuppressive medication

- Have incurable cancers
- Have debilitating diseases that severely limit their life expectancy
- Have severe, disabling psychiatric disease

INHERITED KIDNEY DISEASE

The most common type of inherited kidney disease is autosomal dominant polycystic kidney disease (ADPKD). In this condition, one parent affected with the condition passes it to his or her children. This condition rarely develops without an affected parent. Men and women are equally affected.

With this polycystic kidney disease, the kidneys are a normal size at birth; then they begin to expand due to multiple cysts (fluid-filled sacs) developing in both organs. (See Fig. 2.6) The cysts grow, multiply, and eventually replace healthy kidney tissue. As the number and size of the cysts grows, kidney function declines. Cysts also may appear in other organs, such as the liver, spleen, and uterus. These other cysts rarely cause symptoms or affect body function.

Symptoms

Some with this condition do not have symptoms, and they can expect a normal life span. Others will eventually have kidney failure. Symptoms occur at different times in various people; many do not need dialysis to support their kidneys until they are around 55 years of age. The age of onset of symptoms is usually similar within families.

When symptoms do occur, the most common ones are back and abdominal pain, bloody urine, recurrent

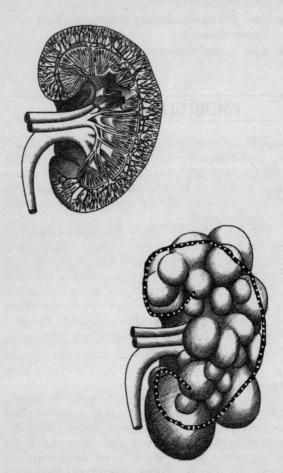

Figure 2.6 Polycystic Kidney Disease
In polycystic kidney disease, the kidneys are normal at birth (left);
but as the individual grows older, they begin to become enlarged
and deformed (right) with fluid-filled sacs, or cysts, that begin to
multiply and eventually replace healthy tissue in the kidney.

urinary tract infections, high blood pressure, or kidney stones. ADPKD is also associated with weakness in the wall of the blood vessels in the brain called cerebral aneurysm. If these aneurysms rupture, it is life-threatening and can be fatal. However, with special X-ray studies, aneurysms usually can be detected before rupture occurs.

Diagnosis

Diagnosis of ADPKD usually depends on detection of the cysts in those who have a family history of the disease. In adults, the enlarged kidneys can be felt on physical exam; other, nonsurgical methods of detection, such as ultrasound, can also detect them. If an ultrasound is done after the age of 30 and cysts are absent, ADPKD is not present. Genetic testing is available to detect the disease even before cysts begin forming, if blood can be obtained from a family member with the disease.

Treatment

People with autosomal dominant polycystic kidney disease should be alert to medical problems, such as high blood pressure and urinary tract infections, that can go along with the disorder and make it worse. Aggressive treatment of these other medical problems may slow the decline in kidney function. Bleeding into the cysts can occur and can be painful. The pain should be treated with painkillers.

Since autosomal dominant polycystic kidney disease is a genetic condition, it can be passed on by either parent to the children. If you have this condition or you have a family history of it, you may want to have genetic counseling.

TUMORS OF THE URINARY SYSTEM

Kidney Tumors

Tumors, or growths, on the kidney can be cystic (fluid-filled) or solid, cancerous or noncancerous. Most kidney tumors do not cause symptoms. When they do, blood may appear in the urine.

Kidney tumors are detected by imaging techniques that allow examining the kidney without surgery. Several examinations may be needed to determine the size of the tumor and whether it has spread outside the kidney or not.

Although a kidney tumor is serious, it can be treated. When a tumor is suspected of being a cancer, the whole kidney can be removed by surgery. (You can live a normal life with just one kidney.) Chemotherapy may be required. With the increased use of imaging techniques today, many kidney tumors are discovered when they are small and have not yet caused symptoms.

Bladder Tumors

Bladder tumors often cause symptoms of urinary frequency or urgency. There also may be visible blood in the urine or blood seen during a microscopic examination of the urine. Most bladder tumors are cancerous; usually they can be easily treated if caught in time. Smoking increases the risk of bladder cancer, sometimes for years after the habit has been stopped.

Most bladder cancers grow from the lining of the bladder and not below the surface of the bladder. These tumors can be treated through a cystoscope; once inserted into the bladder, this small instrument scrapes the tumor off the lining of the bladder. Unfortunately, bladder cancers tend to recur, either at a different place on the bladder lining or along the ureters or in the kidneys. Long-term follow-up care is needed to be sure the cancer has not reappeared. When new tumors are detected early, continued scraping of the bladder lining eventually cures the cancer. If tumors recur often, medication to prevent this can be placed in the bladder through a catheter tube.

If tumors have grown into the wall of the bladder, additional treatment is needed. This may include partial or total removal of the bladder, radiation, or chemotherapy.

SYSTEMIC DISORDERS

Systemic disorders affect the body as a whole. Some have a particular effect on the kidneys and urinary tract. They include diabetes, high blood pressure, sickle cell disease, lupus, and sexually transmitted diseases.

Diabetes Mellitus

Diabetes is a complex metabolic disorder in which the body cannot process glucose. Normally, the pancreas produces insulin to help with the utilization of dietary sugars. If it does not produce enough insulin or if the insulin is ineffective, levels of sugar in the blood increase. Some need insulin injections to keep their blood sugar levels stable, while others can control them by diet, exercise, and pills.

Diabetes also affects other organs such as the heart, brain, nerves, eyes, bladder, and kidneys. Women with diabetes who must take insulin have a substantial risk of developing kidney disease, usually 15–20 years after diabetes starts.

Kidney disease in people with diabetes usually results from the high blood glucose level, causing the nephrons to work too hard (hyperfiltration). Later, increased amounts of protein appear in the urine, and in time the kidneys lose the ability to function. Eventually, kidney failure occurs. In fact, kidney disease due to diabetes is one of the most common causes of end-stage renal disease. Diabetics are also much more likely to have other problems with the urinary system, such as urinary tract infections. Additionally, they may have high blood pressure, poor vision, and heart disease.

Keeping blood glucose at a normal level can help prevent damage to the kidneys as well as other organs. Diabetics can help prevent problems by seeking early care from a specialist, following their doctor's recommendations, and being alert to symptoms and infections. Because women with diabetes often have hypertension, lowering the blood pressure is very important. Taking medications such as ACE inhibitors may delay the development of ESRD, as these medications prevent the kidneys from working too hard and losing their ability to function.

Although dialysis or transplantation can correct many of the complications of kidney failure caused by diabetes, neither can prevent the effects of diabetes on other organs. A transplant may help with kidney function, but diabetes will recur in the transplanted kidney. Pancreas transplants are now in an early stage of development. Successful pancreas transplants remove the need for insulin injections and eliminate the complications of diabetes in other organs.

High Blood Pressure

Kidney disease is often associated with high blood pressure. Diseases of the kidney, such as renal artery stenosis and glomerulonephritis, can cause high blood pressure. Conversely, high blood pressure itself can cause ongoing kidney damage. Detection and treatment of high blood pressure, which may have no symptoms in its early phases, can prevent kidney damage and preserve kidney function.

Sickle Cell Disease

Sickle cell disease is an inherited condition that predominantly affects African-Americans. It also can occur in people of Mediterranean descent. It occurs in two forms, SA (sickle cell trait) and SS (sickle cell disease). SS disease tends to be more severe but less common. Sickle cell disease results when a component of the red blood cells, hemoglobin, is formed abnormally. This causes the red blood cells to curve or "sickle." Sickled cells may block the blood vessels, prevent normal blood circulation, and cause great pain. If the sickled cells become lodged inside the kidneys, they can damage kidney function.

Sickle cell disease can produce severe bleeding in the kidneys, due to the poor blood supply, as well as death of kidney tissue. Glomerulonephritis may also occur, or pieces of kidney tissue may actually break off and be passed like a stone.

Lupus

Systemic lupus erythematosus, or lupus, is more common in women than in men. In this autoimmune disease, the body forms antibodies against its own tissues. It can affect many organs in the body, including the kidneys.

Diagnosis of kidney problems in a woman who has lupus begins with examination of a urine sample. The urine can be completely normal, or there can be protein or red blood cells in it. (Even if a woman has no symptoms and her urine tests are normal, a kidney biopsy can find mild changes.)

There are several types of kidney disease in lupus. Its mildest form may show up as only minimal change in the patient's urinalysis, and is rarely progressive. Some lupus patients develop nephrotic syndrome, and hypertension is common. In its most dangerous form, kidney disease due to lupus causes kidney damage at an accelerated rate.

The treatment of lupus with kidney involvement is complex, often requiring treatment with intravenous steroids and immunosuppressants. Results are variable, so treatment should be started early by an experienced nephrologist.

Sexually Transmitted Diseases

Sexually transmitted diseases (STDs) are infections passed on during sexual intercourse. Some STDs affect the kidneys.

Syphilis

Syphilis has existed for a long time. As with many other STDs, its rates of infection have increased dramatically, especially among African-American women.

Syphilis is caused by infection with an organism known as Treponema pallidum. Its early effects include painless sores around the genitals, fever, sore throat, headache, and a rash. If it is not treated, it can affect many body systems, including the kidneys. When the immune system tries to fight off syphilis, the nephrotic syndrome may result. All patients with the nephrotic syndrome should be tested for both syphilis and HIV. Syphilis can be treated with penicillin.

HIV and AIDS

Infection with human immunodeficiency virus (HIV) usually leads to AIDS, which is a fatal disease, months to years later. Some people infected with HIV develop kidney problems such as nephrotic syndrome or kidney failure. When HIV causes the nephrotic syndrome, it is often associated with focal glomerulonephritis, which in turn tends to cause a rapid form of renal failure. A kidney biopsy can identify this problem.

An infected woman who has kidney failure but has not yet developed AIDS may be a candidate for dialysis. Some women with HIV are well enough so that dialysis can be performed at home, and some who are otherwise well can continue on dialysis for years.

Unfortunately, AIDS-associated kidney disease is more severe and harder to treat than other causes. Uremia usually develops in 3–6 months. General treatment depends largely on the woman's health. If her condition is fairly stable and her quality of life is acceptable to her, she may wish to use dialysis. When AIDS is very advanced, a woman's quality of life is poor and dialysis is unlikely to prolong her life.

Receiving a kidney transplant is not an option for a woman who has either HIV infection or AIDS. Transplantation requires suppressing the immune system so that the kidney is not rejected. This is too risky in someone whose immune system already functions poorly.

PREGNANCY AND THE URINARY TRACT

Although some changes in kidney function normally happen throughout a woman's menstrual cycle—such as premenstrual bloating from fluid retention—the major concern is pregnancy. Many of the changes in the body during pregnancy can affect the kidneys and the rest of the urinary tract. Some of these changes are harmless, but others bear careful watching and may require treatment.

Normal Pregnancy

During pregnancy, your body must produce enough blood to circulate through your own body and also that of the fetus. To do this, the kidneys must work harder and increase in size, and there is salt and water retention. Due to hormonal changes, blood pressure frequently drops slightly in the first trimester of pregnancy and goes back to normal closer to the time of the infant's birth.

The effects of hormones produced in pregnancy and the growing fetus cause the ureters to expand and remain that way for up to 4 months after the baby is born. Although this is a normal development, it can be mistaken for hydronephrosis—a sign of urinary obstruction in women who are not pregnant.

As the uterus grows in pregnancy, it puts pressure on the bladder. For this reason, early in the pregnancy you feel the need to urinate more often. As pregnancy progresses and the uterus sits higher in the abdomen, the pressure on the bladder is eased slightly.

Gradual swelling of the extremities due to fluid retention often occurs in pregnancy, particularly in the last trimester. You may need to buy larger shoes or find that your rings are too tight. This usually disappears soon after the baby is born. Minor swelling is not usually a concern, but swelling that causes substantial weight gain of more than 1 pound per week or rising blood pressure is dangerous and should be treated.

Urinary Tract Conditions in Pregnancy

Some conditions that affect the urinary tract are more common in pregnancy. Others can affect the pregnancy and endanger the fetus if they are not carefully monitored and treated.

Urinary Tract Infections

Women are at greater risk for developing a urinary tract infection when they are pregnant. Even if you have never had such an infection before, you may develop one when pregnant. The exact reason for this is unknown, but it is thought that hormonal changes and the effect of the uterus pressing on the urinary tract are responsible.

If a urinary tract infection in pregnancy goes untreated, it can cause several problems, including severe infection, premature labor, and fetal death. For this reason, visits to an obstetrician include tests for detecting urinary tract infections. If infection does occur, it should be treated promptly with antibiotics.

High Blood Pressure

Normally, blood pressure drops somewhat in pregnancy. If blood pressure rises instead, it causes risks for the woman and fetus alike. In fact, high blood pressure is the second largest cause of maternal deaths in pregnancy. The fetus may be born too early, may be too small, or may be stillborn. Proper care of high blood pressure in pregnancy is essential.

If you had high blood pressure before you became pregnant, you need special care by both an obstetrician specializing in high-risk care and a hypertension specialist. Some medications used for treating blood pressure can harm the fetus, and so treatment should be selected carefully. For example, ACE inhibitors should not be used by pregnant women. If you suffer from mild hypertension, you may find the dip in blood pressure early in pregnancy beneficial. Your doctor may be able to taper off your medication, but careful monitoring is still required. Blood pressure may rise late in pregnancy and require treatment again.

High blood pressure can occur in pregnancy even if a woman did not have it before. Pregnancy-induced hypertension, preeclampsia and eclampsia, is more likely to occur in:

- Women with kidney disease
- Women with a family history of the condition
- Older women who have not had children before
- Women carrying twins
- Women with an immune system disorder, such as lupus

When pregnant women with high blood pressure excrete too much protein in their urine, particularly in the latter half of pregnancy, it is called preeclampsia. A woman with preeclampsia can develop kidney failure, bleeding, and a complication called eclampsia, in which the brain is affected and seizures occur. This is very dangerous and may cause death.

If blood pressure reaches dangerous levels late in pregnancy, when the fetus is mature and healthy enough to live on its own, prompt delivery of the baby can save both mother and child. When blood pressure increases earlier in pregnancy, before the fetus can survive on its own, treatment depends on how high the blood pressure is. Small increases can generally be monitored by the doctor without treatment. More severe increases may need to be treated with antihypertensive drugs. If the increase is very high, the baby may have to be delivered to save the mother's life.

After delivery, a woman's blood pressure usually returns to normal. In some hypertensive women, however, it may remain high, requiring drugs. Since antihypertensive medication is excreted in breast milk, breastfeeding may not be possible.

Pregnancy in Women with Kidney Disease

It is not always clear how the added stress of pregnancy may affect the kidneys in a woman whose kidneys are already functioning poorly. It depends on the type and extent of the kidney disease, as well as how poorly the kidneys are working. Women with mild kidney disease generally do well and are not likely to have long-term problems. Still, all women with kidney disease who become pregnant should be treated by both a nephrologist and an obstetrician specializing in high-risk pregnancies.

Most women with some degree of kidney failure have an increased risk of high blood pressure, preeclampsia, and eclampsia if they become pregnant. Women with lupus or diabetes are prone to kidney problems during pregnancy. Some moderate kidney problems can worsen if the woman becomes pregnant.

Women with severe kidney failure may find it difficult to become pregnant. If they do conceive, their pregnancies can be risky, and usually result in a premature birth. Women who are on dialysis may be able to become pregnant but require almost daily dialysis. Commonly, the pregnancy ends in miscarriage. For these reasons, women with severe kidney conditions are usually discouraged from becoming pregnant.

On the other hand, pregnant women who have had a kidney transplant often do quite well. However, they require special care involving the transplant team and the obstetrician.

DIAGNOSTIC TECHNIQUES FOR URINARY PROBLEMS

History and Physical Exam

As with other conditions, the diagnosis of a disorder of the urinary system begins with the doctor or nurse taking your medical history and performing a physical exam. Be prepared to describe your family history, your symptoms, previous urinary tract conditions, type of diet, and so on. You may find it helpful to keep a diary of when symptoms occur and what seems to provoke them. The physical exam allows the doctor or nurse to check the strength of the pelvic floor muscles.

Usually the doctor's diagnosis is based on the results of the history, the physical exam, and specific tests. Laboratory tests, biopsies (taking samples of tissue for study), and special imaging methods for looking at the kidneys and the bladder are used.

Urinalysis

Urinalysis is the most basic test performed. It involves obtaining a clean specimen of urine and can provide much information about the function of the kidneys and bladder.

A clean specimen cannot be contaminated with blood or other substances from the vagina. Providing a clean catch urine specimen requires you to follow these four steps:

1. Wash your hands.
2. Hold your labia (lips surrounding the vagina) open and clean the area with an antiseptic towelette.

3. Void the first part of the urine stream into the toilet.
4. Catch part of the rest of the flow into a sterile cup.

If you are menstruating, you should insert a tampon into the vagina before following the steps for providing a urine specimen. Alternatively, a clean urine sample can be obtained by catheterization. A doctor or nurse places a thin tube called a catheter through the urethra up into the bladder. A sample is obtained, and the tube is withdrawn. Catheterization is a simple but not routine way of obtaining urine.

A clean sample of urine is necessary for many tests. Laboratory tests for electrolytes and other substances normally in the urine can provide much information about how well the kidneys are working. Other tests that may be done include:

- Chemical testing for sugar, protein, blood, bacteria, and pH (acidity)
- Examination under a microscope for red blood cells (a sign of bleeding) or white blood cells and bacteria (a sign of infection)

Urine Culture

In a urine culture, a portion of the clean sample is poured on a culture plate or the plate is dipped into the sample. After allowing time for growth of the bacteria, the colonies on the plate are counted. A significant colony count denotes infection. The infecting bacteria are tested for sensitivity to a number of antibiotics, so the appropriate medication can be chosen.

Kidney Biopsy

In a biopsy, a small sample of tissue is taken from the kidney for study. With many conditions, this is the only way to make a diagnosis. In most women, a biopsy is a fairly simple procedure that can be done with local anesthesia by a nephrologist. Kidney ultrasound is used to verify the exact location of the biopsy site, and a small sample is withdrawn through a needle. The kidney tissue is looked at under several different kinds of microscopes. This provides the most accurate description of the kidney's anatomy.

The amount of tissue taken for a biopsy is so small that it does not affect the kidney's function. After a biopsy, you may have microscopic blood in your urine for a few days afterward. The risks of the procedure are low when performed by an experienced nephrologist, and biopsies are usually safe even for older women. However, complications can occur, including severe bleeding, infection, and even loss of the kidney. For safety, the nephrologist performs blood and urine tests and scans before the biopsy. After having a biopsy, you should rest for a day and avoid strenuous activity and exercise for about 2 weeks.

Imaging Techniques

There are different techniques currently arvailable to determine the anatomy and function of the kidney. Your physician will select the imaging technique based on the information needed in your situation.

Intravenous Pyelography

Pyelography creates a picture of the kidneys and ureters. A special dye that shows up on the X-ray is injected into a vein. The dye filters through the kidneys and is excreted into the ureters and the bladder. This allows detection of kidney stones, infection, tumors, and obstructions.

This test is not done in women allergic to the dye used in these studies or in pregnant women.

Ultrasound

Ultrasound is the use of sound waves to create a picture of an organ or area of body. A small device called a transducer is rubbed over the outside of the body near the area to be studied. Sound waves bounce off the organ or area and form a picture that is displayed on a monitor. Ultrasound can be used to examine the kidney, ureters, and bladder.

Ultrasound can be used by persons who cannot tolerate the dye in pyelography. The sound waves do not harm a fetus, so ultrasound is safely used in pregnancy.

Computerized Axial Tomography

A computerized axial tomography, or CT, scan is a type of X-ray that can create a picture of the abdominal organs, including the kidneys, ureters, and bladder. It is effective in showing tumors, stones, and some problems with blood vessels.

The best pictures result when a woman having a CT scan both ingests special material that appears on the picture and has similar material injected. However, in women with kidney failure, especially those with diabetes, the injection often worsens function and is not recommended. Pregnant women should avoid CT scans because of the risk to the fetus.

Magnetic Resonance Imaging

Magnetic resonance imaging, or MRI, uses magnetic waves instead of special contrast material to create a picture. Although safe for most women, it is usually reserved for those who cannot use CT. In some kidney conditions, MRI will produce a better picture of soft tissue than CT.

Cystoscopy

During cystoscopy, the inside of the bladder is examined with a small, telescopelike instrument that is passed through the urethra into the bladder. The exam is done with local anesthesia, and most women tolerate it well. Because a woman's urethra is shorter than a man's, she is likely to find this examination more comfortable than a man would. When the inside of the urethra is examined at the same time, this is referred to as cystourethroscopy. Cystoscopy and cystourethroscopy can detect many problems in the urinary tract, including tumors, obstructions, and fistulas. Fistulas are small openings in the bladder, ureters, or urethra that allow urine to leak out.

Urodynamics

Urodynamics is the study of how the bladder functions. One type of urodynamics is cystometry, the study of how the bladder's pressure is affected by the amount of urine it contains. At its most basic, cystometry involves placing a catheter up the urethra into the bladder. Sterile saline solution (salt water) is instilled into the bladder through the catheter to mimic the effect of urine in the bladder. Special equipment measures the pressure changes in the bladder as it fills.

This test can give information about the bladder's capacity. Normal bladder capacity is about one pint. If a woman's bladder does not hold enough urine, she is at risk for urinary incontinence or infection.

The main use for this test, though, is to measure how the bladder and the urethra react to different volumes of fluid. Measurements of their ability to stretch and contract can be made. If these measurements are made while a woman coughs, jumps, or squats, it provides an idea of how well the system performs under stress. This technique is important in evaluating urinary incontinence.

WHERE TO GET MORE INFORMATION

Many conditions affecting the urinary tract can be long-term chronic problems. Fortunately, many groups can provide both information and support:

■ **The Interstitial Cystitis Association,** established by women who have this condition, has been an important influence in increasing the amount of research money dedicated to discovering a cause and cure for this often-debilitating problem. For more information, contact the Interstitial Cystitis Association, PO Box 1553, Madison Square Station, New York, NY 10159; 800-422-1626.

■ **Help for Incontinent People (HIP), Inc.,** and **The Simon Foundation** provide help to women who have problems with bladder control. Contact Help for Incontinent People, Inc., PO Box 544, Union, SC 29379; 800-BLADDER (800-252-3337). Contact the Simon Foundation, PO Box 835, Wilmette, IL 60091; 800-23SIMON (800-237-4666).

■ **National Kidney Foundation** supports kidney research and works as an advocate for people with kidney disease. It produces educational booklets, sponsors meetings, and provides support groups for patients and their families. Contact the National Kidney Foundation, 30 East 33rd Street, New York, NY 10016; 800-622-9010.

■ **United Network of Organ Sharing** oversees all donations of organs and organ transplants. It also establishes and enforces regulations to ensure equality in organ transplantation and fairness in distribution of donor organs. Call 804-330-8500.

Books are another good source for information. Except as noted, many of these books can be found at a local library:

■ Rebecca Chalker and Kristine E. Whitmore, *Overcoming Bladder Disorders* (New York: Harper and Row, 1990).

■ Kathryn L. Burgio, K. Lynette Peace, and Angelo J. Lucio, *Staying Dry—A Guide to Bladder Control* (Baltimore, MD: Johns Hopkins University Press, 1989).

■ Katherine Jeter, Nancy Faller, and Christine Norton, *Nursing for Incontinence* (Philadelphia, PA: Harcourt Brace Jovanovich, 1990).

■ Pauline E. Chiarelli, *Women's Waterworks—Curing Incontinence* is available from Help for Incontinent People.

■ Lisa Delaney with Cemela Longon, *Managing Urinary Incontinence: A Patient's Guide* can be requested from the Agency for Health Care Policy and Research by calling 800-358-9295.

PART III
The Digestive System

Susan Cobb Stewart, M.D., F.A.C.P.

The act of consuming and digesting food may appear simple, but it's actually a complex process that involves a number of finely coordinated chemical and mechanical reactions of the upper and lower gastrointestinal tract. The digestive system consists of many organs that are connected to each other, so our very survival depends on the smooth functioning of each component. It's easy to see why our entire outlook on life changes when some element of the system goes awry.

STRUCTURE AND FUNCTION

Each part of the gastrointestinal system has its own role to play in the digestion and absorption of food and the elimination of waste. (See Fig. 3.1) The major organs are the following:

- *The esophagus*, a muscular tube that connects the bottom of the throat (pharynx) with the stomach.

- *The stomach*, a pear-shaped, muscular organ situated mostly on the left-hand side below the ribs. The stomach is lined with special cells that produce acid and digestive enzymes that break down food.

- *The small intestine*, which in an adult is about 22 feet long. It consists of the *duodenum*, a short portion immediately beyond the stomach that is the place of entry for ducts coming from the liver and pancreas; the *jejunum*, the long portion of the small intestine that follows the duodenum and is lined with specialized cells that assist in diluting, digesting, and absorbing nutrients; and the *ileum*, the long portion of the small intestine that follows the jejunum and is primarily involved in absorbing nutrients and water.

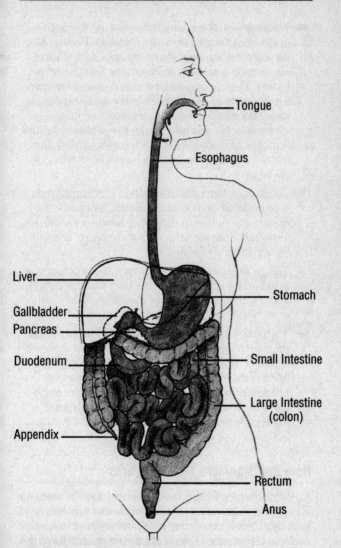

Figure 3.1 Anatomy of the Digestive System

- *The large intestine*, which receives all the undigested food, water, and other intestinal waste. It includes the *cecum* (where the appendix is located), which is part of the *colon*, the final 6 feet of bowel. The colon extracts much of the water from the contents of the stomach and transforms the liquid mass into solid waste, or feces. The waste material is eliminated through the *rectum*—the last 8 inches of the colon—and the *anus*, a muscular tube containing the sphincter muscles that control elimination.

- *The liver*, a large organ located in the upper right side of the abdomen, has multiple functions: it manufactures bile to digest fat, processes nutrients absorbed from the intestine, and extracts and eliminates drugs and toxins.

- *The gallbladder* is a small, pouchlike structure that is linked by ducts to both the liver and the duodenum. The main function of the gallbladder is to store bile from the liver.

- *The pancreas*, a glandular organ that branches off the intestinal tract and contains cells that make enzymes to digest fat, protein, and carbohydrate from consumed food. Two important hormones are produced by the pancreas, insulin and glucagon. Each is essential in the metabolism of carbohydrates.

How the Digestive System Works

Digestion begins in the mouth, where food is chewed and mixed with saliva, which contains enzymes and fluid that break down the food and make it easier to swallow. The semisolid food mass then passes down the esophagus into the stomach. The stomach responds by secreting hydrochloric acid and a protein-digesting enzyme called pepsin for a period of 3 to 4 hours. The stomach muscles mix the food with the secretions, breaking it down further. The stomach then releases small amounts of the food, now liquid containing fine particles, into the duodenum.

The presence of fat in the duodenum initiates the release of secretin, a gastrointestinal hormone that slows down the muscular activity of the stomach and causes the food to be retained in the stomach until adequate digestive enzymes are available to break down the fat. Cells in the wall of the duodenum, sensing the composition of the food, also secrete cholecystokinin, another hormone that, together with secretin, stimulates the liver and pancreas to release digestive enzymes and bile. Complex molecules of carbohydrate, fat, and protein are then broken down into sugars, simple fats, and amino acids that are absorbed through the cells lining the jejunum.

The ileum, the last part of the small intestine, absorbs the fluids and bile acids so these chemicals can be returned to the liver and reused. By the time the food is ready to pass into the large intestine, almost all of its nutrients have been absorbed.

The role of the large intestine is to process the undigested food, fiber, and water coming from the small intestine. This liquid, called chyme, enters the colon and is dehydrated by the colon cells. Mucus from those cells and bacteria that inhabit the colon are added to the chyme. (The bacteria break down some of the dietary fiber that is not digested by the stomach or small intestine.) As the liquid mass moves across and down the colon, it becomes progressively more solid and turns into what we call *feces* or stool.

The reflex to defecate, or get rid of the feces, is initiated by the entry of stool into the rectum. Once the brain is signaled, the internal sphincter muscles relax.

The brain retains control over the external sphincter, however, and ultimately makes the decision whether defecation takes place. The defecation reflex can also be signaled by the entry of food into the stomach; this is known as the gastrocolic reflex.

COMMON DIGESTIVE SYMPTOMS

We all occasionally develop minor digestive problems that are self-limiting in nature and usually clear up with time. If the symptoms persist, consult a physician.

Gastrointestinal Pain

Stomachache is probably the single most frequent reason for consulting a doctor. But the stomach is the culprit in only a small percentage of cases. Because the gastrointestinal tract shares the abdominal cavity with organs of other systems, the pain could be originating from the spleen (left upper quadrant), the kidneys (mid-abdomen), the bladder (lower abdomen), or the reproductive organs—the ovaries, fallopian tubes, and uterus—(lower abdomen). (See Fig. 3.2)

Nausea and Vomiting

From time to time everyone experiences a queasy feeling in the pit of the stomach—nausea—and the forceful and uncontrolled expelling, or vomiting, of food. Centers in the brain coordinate the following events: nausea is felt in the back of the throat, the chest, or the upper abdomen; the salivary glands are stimulated to release saliva; the sphincters in the esophagus relax and the pyloric sphincter contracts; the muscles of the stomach contract violently and force the contents of the stomach up the esophagus and out the mouth.

The vomiting reflex is a complex reaction that can be initiated by a variety of causes. The stimuli from the brain may be psychological, such as a terrible sight or smell. Or there may be direct stimulation from the balance centers of the inner ear, as occurs in motion sickness. Other causes are the morning sickness of pregnancy, irritation of the stomach by an infectious agent or a chemical irritant such as alcohol, and stimulation of the back of the throat, which induces gagging and, perhaps, vomiting. More serious reasons for vomiting are an inflammation of an organ adjacent to the stomach, such as the pancreas or gallbladder, blockage of the outlet of the stomach (the pylorus), and a blockage of the intestine, usually from a tumor.

Vomiting must be distinguished from *regurgitation*, which is the sudden reflux of recently ingested food to the mouth without accompanying nausea or any particular cause. Regurgitation also can occur when there is blockage of the esophagus, usually by a stricture or a tumor. In this situation, the food cannot enter the stomach and simply comes back up. The syndrome of reflux esophagitis, in which the sphincter between the stomach and the esophagus is incompetent, also causes regurgitation. Another type of regurgitation, called rumination, is common to the digestive processes of cattle and related animals, and has been described in some people. Rumination is the regurgitation of partially digested food, which is then chewed and reswallowed. Finally, people suffering from the eating disorders anorexia nervosa and/or bulimia often rid themselves of unwanted consumed food by inducing vomiting or learning how to periodically regurgiate food from the stomach.

Important symptoms, when medical attention should be sought, include severe and persistent vomiting, vomiting blood, and vomiting accompanied by persistent abdominal pain.

Heartburn and Indigestion

Most people have experienced heartburn at some time in their lives, and women may experience it frequently in pregnancy. Heartburn is a burning sensation that arises behind the breastbone. A component of indigestion, heartburn is caused by the reflux of stomach acid into the esophagus and usually occurs after a heavy meal.

The general discomfort that can occur after eating is called indigestion, or dyspepsia. Symptoms include a

Figure 3.2   Sources of Abdominal Pain
Upper abdominal pain: Pain coming from the lower esophagus, the stomach, the duodenum, and the pancreas is usually felt in the mid portion of the upper abdomen. Gallbladder pain is felt on the right side and sometimes radiates around to the back. Pain from the spleen is on the left side. Kidney pain is sometimes felt in the upper abdomen but more often localizes to the back just below the lowest ribs.

Midabdominal pain: Pain from the small intestine is felt around the navel, called "periumbilical." It is often due to distention of bowel loops by gas, either from food eaten or because there is a blockage of the bowel, often caused by adhesions formed after surgery. Pain from a kidney stone in the ureter can be felt here and radiates down toward the vulva.

Lower abdominal pain: Distention and inflammation of the colon are felt in the lower abdomen, even though parts of the colon are located in the upper and mid portions of the abdomen. Appendicitis is felt in the right lower abdomen; diverticulitis on the left. In women, pain from the ovary or the fallopian tube is located on left or right; pain from the uterus or the bladder in the middle of the lower abdomen.

gnawing discomfort in the upper abdomen, bloating, nausea, and gas. Some people experience chronic indigestion, but in most cases it is a benign disorder and disappears on its own. The causes of indigestion include eating too fast or too heavily, and stress. You may get relief by modifying your diet, stopping smoking, eating more regular, smaller meals, and reducing the stress in your life. Avoid drinking caffeinated beverages or too much alcohol, and taking excessive amounts of aspirin, which can cause irritation of the stomach lining.

Important symptoms, when you should seek the attention of a physician, include persistent indigestion, and severe stomach pain that lasts for a few hours or wakes you up at night.

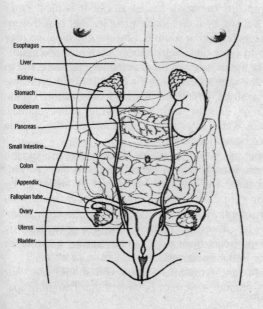

Lower Intestinal Problems: Diarrhea, Bloating, and Constipation

Diarrhea is defined as any change in bowel habit that involves an increase in frequency or a change in consistency of the stool from solid to loose. Diarrhea can be the result of an infection or irritation in the intestines, the ingestion of a nonabsorbable substance that forces the intestine to hold extra water (lactose intolerance), or a disease in the bowel itself. The characteristics most important to note are frequency of bowel movements, duration of the diarrhea, and whether it is accompanied by vomiting, fever, pain, or bleeding. If you suffer from acute diarrhea, make sure you replace the lost fluids to avoid dehydration.

Constipation refers to a change in bowel habit that results in less frequent, harder stools. It is most commonly caused by a diet inadequate in fiber or a disruption of regular diet or routine. Chronic constipation may be due to poor diet, dehydration, certain medications, stress, or the pressure of other activities that force you to ignore the urge to evacuate the bowel. Avoid excessive use of laxatives, which may lead to a dependence on the medication. Exercise, eating lots of fruits and vegetables, adequate water intake, and fiber in the diet usually improve bowel function.

Bloating is an occasional enlargement of the abdomen, usually due to excessive gas in the gastrointestinal tract. The gas can be caused by smoking, by chewing gum, by drinking carbonated beverages, or by the consumption of certain foods. More seriously, bloating can be caused by a partial blockage of the tract by adhesions (scars from prior surgery) or by a tumor or stricture in the intestines.

Important symptoms—when you should see your doctor—include severe or persistent diarrhea, constipation, or bloating, and especially the appearance of blood in the stool. Blood in the stool may indicate tears of the anus or ulcerated hemorrhoids, but also can be a symptom of inflammatory bowel disease (IBD) or cancer of the colon.

Where Does It Hurt?

If you experience a pain in your abdominal area, it helps in the diagnosis to know the specific area of distress and the organ that may be causing it.

Upper abdomen: Lower esophagus, stomach, duodenum, liver, gallbladder, pancreas, spleen, kidney

Mid-abdomen: Small intestine

Lower abdomen: Colon, appendix (right side), ovaries (both sides), fallopian tubes, uterus, and bladder (center)

General, diffuse pain all over the abdomen usually reflects the distention of multiple organs—stomach, small intestine, large intestine—or irritation of the peritoneum, the lining of the abdominal cavity. It is also important to take note of the characteristics of the pain, which will help your doctor narrow down the diagnostic possibilities and determine which tests should be performed. Pay special attention to the following aspects of the pain:

- *Location*. Is the pain in the upper, middle, or lower abdomen? Or is it general and diffuse, over the abdominal area? Does the pain stay in the same area, or does it shoot to another location?

- *Type*. Is the pain sharp or a deep, dull ache? How severe is it?

- *Timing*. Does the pain occur at night only, or during the day? How often? Was it sudden, or did it develop gradually?

- *Relationship to meals.* Is the pain better after eating, or worse? Does it occur on an empty stomach? After eating certain foods?
- *Response to treatment.* Are there medications that seem to alleviate the pain?
- *Relationship to stress.* Does the pain occur after an emotional upset or a difficult day?

HOW TO PREVENT DIGESTIVE PROBLEMS

The maxim "We are what we eat" could be changed to "We feel what we eat" when it comes to the digestive system. The foods we eat, the liquids we drink, the drugs we take, all can affect the internal workings of the gastrointestinal tract for better or for worse. Overindulgence in food and drink can especially affect our digestive system adversely, leading to indigestion, heartburn, regurgitation, excess gas, and bloating.

The Healthy Woman's Diet

Regularity and a selectivity in food and drink pay off in a healthy gut—especially in the middle years, when many digestive problems are apt to show up. The "iron" stomach of youth—when you could eat anything—is but a memory. It's necessary to take a good, hard look at your eating habits, and change them gradually and permanently to fit a new, healthier lifestyle. A new eating program might include the following suggestions:

- *Eat regularly, but not too well.* In our society, where food is generally plentiful, the consequences of overeating are all around us.

Americans have a high rate of obesity, from both eating too much and too often, from eating excessively fatty foods, and from not exercising. There are other factors, besides the availability of food, that prompt us to overeat. The sensitive neural and hormonal mechanisms that tell us we have eaten enough are constantly being disrupted by such cultural overrides as the "clean plate syndrome" (drilled into us by our parents), too large servings in restaurants, the use of food as a bribe or reward, and the urging of TV food ads to eat, eat, eat.

■ Generally, however, our custom of three meals a day—breakfast, lunch, and dinner—works well with the basic physiology of the human intestinal tract. The stomach processes a meal in about 4 to 6 hours. When digestion begins, cells lining the stomach and intestines release gastrointestinal hormones that stimulate the gallbladder, the liver, the pancreas, the intestines, and the brain. These hormones keep the organs functioning and healthy.

■ *Don't overload at one meal.* Eating too much at a meal causes pain from the stretching of the stomach walls, as well as the possibility of regurgitation of food into the esophagus. It may help to eat only half of what is on your plate, or wait 20 minutes before taking a second helping.

■ *Avoid eating between meals.* This is often where the calories mount up and the fat collects. If you must have a snack, make it a nutritious one: fresh fruit or raw vegetables. Especially avoid eating when you are doing something else—like watching TV—because it is harder to detect the "I'm full" signals from the body when your attention is distracted.

■ *Eat the right foods.* Nutrition is powerful medicine. Today, it's common knowledge that a diet includ-

ing certain foods may increase the risk of disease,
and a variety of other foods may reduce it. It's also
important to reduce your total fat intake to 30 percent or less of your total calories. Eat 5 or more
servings of vegetables and fruits every day, and
keep your protein intake down. And eat lots of
fiber.

■ *Exercise regularly.* Just changing your diet isn't
enough. It's vital to go out every day and exercise.
Walk briskly, swing your arms, and breathe deeply.
If you are up to it, and your doctor approves, start
a jogging program or aerobic exercises. Join a
health club. If you don't have the time, make the
time. Once you begin to exercise, you'll feel better, look better, have an improved outlook on life
(all those endorphins!), and feel more in control.
The key is regularity and increasing your speed,
duration, and length of exercise *gradually*, not in
spurts.

■ *Avoid too much alcohol.* If you want to be good to
your digestive system, don't drink to excess.
Alcohol can inflict serious damage on the digestive organs, including cancer of the esophagus,
bleeding of the stomach wall, ulcers in the stomach and duodenum, severe inflammation and/or
chronic destruction of the pancreas, and scarring
of the liver (cirrhosis). If your doctor tells you that
your digestive problems may be a result of too
much drinking, you must seriously address the
question of why you drink and whether you have
lost control over your intake of alcohol. A person
who has a serious medical problem caused by
drinking alcohol and is unable to stop drinking is
very likely to be suffering from alcoholism. The
successful control of alcoholism not only results
in greater health for the digestive system but also

leads to improved life functioning and better inter-
personal relationships.

■ *Don't smoke.* The list of ill effects on the body
from smoking is lengthy, and the digestive system
is not spared. Smokers have a higher incidence of
stomach and duodenum ulcers. Cancers in the
organs of the upper digestive tract—esophagus,
stomach, pancreas—are more likely in smokers.

Why Fiber Is Important

Your choice of food can determine whether your digestive system works well or gives you trouble. Studies have
shown that the human gastrointestinal system is pro-
grammed to process foods high in undigestible fiber,
such as vegetables, fruits, and the bran part of grains.
Unfortunately, the diet in the United States and many
European countries has eliminated fiber in favor of
processed foods and the overconsumption of meat. If
you habitually choose a hamburger for lunch instead of
a salad, or ice cream rather than an apple, you are
choosing a low-fiber diet.

The consequences of a low-fiber diet are many and
long-term. Some people may not seem to suffer any
immediate problems, but others may experience constipation, diarrhea, stomach upsets, indigestion, and
bloating. A more serious effect is the slow transit time of
low-fiber foods through the colon. This means that the
contents of the intestine—food residues, products of
digestive juices, bacteria—remain in contact with the
cell lining of the large intestine for a longer period of
time. If the diet is high in fat, as a low-fiber diet often is,
the intestinal contents will be high in bile derivatives,
which can break down into cancer-causing compounds.
In addition, a colon receiving low amounts of fiber re-

quires more muscular activity and pressure to push the contents through; as a result, little out-pouchings called diverticula can develop and cause a serious intestinal disease called diverticulitis.

The best diet for optimal colonic function contains about 20 grams of fiber per day, roughly the amount of fiber in three to five servings of fresh fruit and four servings of vegetables per day, and whole-grain breads and cereals. The advantages of a high-fiber diet are many. Bulkier foods take time to eat and fill the stomach, allowing time for satiety signals to reach the brain. High-fiber foods are lower in fat, so the stomach empties more easily and quickly, and there is less tendency for the formation of gas and bloating, belching, and regurgitation of food. Less fat in the diet also results in less fat and cholesterol in the blood, thus decreasing the risk of coronary disease. A smaller amount of bile is released, reducing the risk of colon polyps and cancer. Finally, because there is less abdominal straining with a high-fiber diet, there is less risk of formation of diverticula in the colon or hemorrhoids around the anal canal.

Cancer Screening of the Digestive System

Cancers of the organs of the digestive system are solid, slow-growing tumors that, once established, are very difficult to treat. Unfortunately, many are not discovered until they have invaded adjacent structures of the body. At the present time, the only gastrointestinal tumor amenable to screening is cancer of the colon. Beginning at age 50, you should have a fecal occult blood test every year and a flexible sigmoidoscopy every 5 years.

If You Have to See Your Doctor

An occasional bout of indigestion, heartburn, nausea, or diarrhea is generally self-limiting and clears up on its own, but there are instances when a digestive problem calls for prompt medical attention.

If you visit your doctor with a digestive complaint, she or he will ask for a detailed history of your problem,

DIGESTIVE SYSTEM SPECIALISTS

When you are suffering from a gastrointestinal ailment, the first person you should see is your primary physician. If the problem cannot be easily resolved, the primary physician will refer you to a gastroenterologist, an internist with advanced specialty training in diseases of the digestive system. She or he can do a number of procedures to diagnose and treat your illness. Other digestive specialists are listed below:

- *Hepatologist.* A specialist in diseases of the liver. A clinical hepatologist is an internist with subspecialty training in gastroenterology, often with advanced research and clinical training in liver disease.

- *Colorectal surgeon.* A surgeon with general surgery training and advanced specialty training in diagnosis and treatment of diseases of the colon, rectum, and anus.

- *Proctologist.* A general term applied to a physician, usually a surgeon, with training and practice expertise in the conditions of the anus and rectum.

and question you about your digestive functions and diet. You will receive a physical evaluation including an abdominal and rectal checkup, and a spot check for hidden blood in the stool. If your symptoms or the exam suggests a particular problem, you may be asked to undergo certain diagnostic tests. Don't be afraid to ask the doctor questions. Why is the test being offered? What does the doctor suspect? What might the test show? What treatment would be recommended on the basis of the test findings? If you are offered medication, ask how the drug works and about any potential side effects.

DISORDERS OF THE ESOPHAGUS

When you eat, the food passes from the back of your mouth into the esophagus, a muscular tube approximately 10 inches long that leads directly into your stomach. While the esophagus moves food along, it must

---

ESOPHAGEAL DISORDERS CAUSING DYSPHAGIA

- Peptic stricture (see Reflux, below)
- Cancer
- Motility disorders
  Spasm
  Scleroderma
  Achalasia
- Neurological disorders
  Myasthenia gravis
  Amyotrophic lateral sclerosis (ALS)

---

also stop material from backing up and reentering the throat (regurgitation) and prevent, at the other end, the backing up of stomach acids into its interior. Two sphincter muscles—one at each end—perform this duty.

Dysphagia

Dysphagia, or difficulty in swallowing, is the most important esophageal symptom. It may indicate an active disease in the lining of the esophagus, faulty muscular action of the esophagus, or a physical obstruction that is blocking the passage of food and/or liquids.

This symptom always merits a visit to the doctor.

Symptoms
The important characteristics of dysphagia are difficulty and pain in swallowing, regurgitation of food, and heartburn.

Aphagia, the complete inability to swallow even saliva, is a medical emergency and requires immediate medical attention.

Causes
Difficulty in swallowing may have various causes, including obstruction by stricture or tumor, or the less common motility disorders and nerve diseases. In any case, a diagnosis is always called for, and physician evaluation should be promptly sought. (See Fig. 3.3)

Reflux Esophagitis, or Gastroesophogeal Reflux Disease (GERD)

When the sphincter separating the stomach from the esophagus becomes weak or fails to function, the acid content of the stomach can wash backward, or "reflux," into the esophagus. The lining of the esophagus can become inflamed or irritated by this acidic fluid, sometimes to the point of ulceration. A serious long-term consequence is esophageal stricture, also called peptic stricture, in which the esophagus becomes severely narrowed and swallowing becomes difficult. Rarely the cells lining the end of the esophagus can change form, a condition called Barrett's esophagus. This condition carries a high risk for the development of cancer of the esophagus. (See Fig. 3.3A & B)

Certain conditions will cause or exacerbate reflux, including pregnancy, weight gain, the wearing of tight

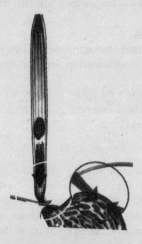

Figure 3.3A Esophageal "Peptic Stricture"
Acid and pepsin in the gastric juice can cause erosions, ulcers, and finally scar formation and thickening of the wall of the lower esophagus, leading to a narrowed area called a stricture. The first symptom is usually difficulty in swallowing solid food, like meat or bread. If the stricture becomes extremely narrow, even liquids cannot pass it. Strictures can be opened by dilators of gradually increasing size, called bougies.

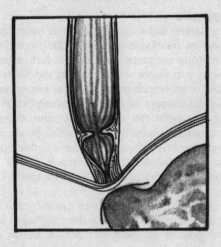

Figure 3.3B Esophageal Ring
Sometimes dysphagia (difficulty in swallowing) is caused by a thin ring of esophageal tissue called a ring or a web. Often this ring is disrupted just by passing the fiberoptic endoscope to investigate the cause of dysphagia. Sometime dilatation with bougies is required to open the ring.

clothing, and straining during bowel movements. Specific chemicals or hormones can relax the gastroesophageal sphincter, such as estrogen (as in pregnancy), caffeine, and nicotine.

Symptoms

The most common symptom is heartburn, a burning sensation usually centered in the chest, although pain can occur in the upper abdomen, the back, or even the neck. Heartburn usually occurs within an hour after a meal; it can also strike at night, while you are lying in bed. Serious complications can result from night reflux if the stomach content enters the lungs, and causes nocturnal asthma or aspiration pneumonia.

Diagnosis

The doctor can make a diagnosis based on your symptoms of heartburn and prescribe accordingly. If your symptoms are particularly severe, further tests may be necessary to discover the cause of the reflux. Often heartburn is accompanied by a *hiatal hernia*, an anatomical displacement of the uppermost portion of the stomach through the diaphragm. The esophageal sphincter and the opening in the diaphragm are normally at the same level, thus producing an added pressure to keep food contents in the stomach. If you have a hiatal hernia, the reflux can occur more easily. (See Fig 3.4)

An X-ray test, called an upper gastrointestinal series (UGIS), can reveal strictures of the esophagus and the size and position of the hiatal hernia. Reflux can be demonstrated by this exam. An *endoscopy* of the esophagus and the stomach can show inflammation and ulceration of the esophageal lining as well as the presence of a hiatal hernia. Biopsies can reveal the extent of damage or the presence of Barrett's changes. *PH monitoring studies* can show if acid is in the esophagus, how often it occurs, and how long the acid remains in the esophagus. There is little to be gained from doing these ancillary diagnostic procedures unless a complication is suspected.

Sometimes there is no relationship between a person's symptoms and the findings of the diagnostic studies. You may find you have a severe peptic stricture, for example, and never recall experiencing heartburn or chest pain. Another person, suffering from severe heartburn and pain, may have a perfectly normal esophageal lining with little inflammation and no stricture.

Treatment

Pharmacological, physiological, physical, and sometimes surgical measures are used to treat reflux.

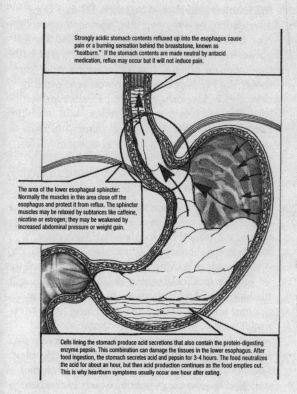

Strongly acidic stomach contents refluxed up into the esophagus cause pain or a burning sensation behind the breaststone, known as "heartburn." If the stomach contents are made neutral by antacid medication, reflux may occur but it will not induce pain.

The area of the lower esophageal sphincter: Normally the muscles in this area close off the esophagus and protect it from reflux. The sphincter muscles may be relaxed by subtances like caffeine, nicotine or estrogen; they may be weakened by increased abdominal pressure or weight gain.

Cells lining the stomach produce acid secretions that also contain the protein-digesting enzyme pepsin. This combination can damage the tissues in the lower esophagus. After food ingestion, the stomach secretes acid and pepsin for 3-4 hours. The food neutralizes the acid for about an hour, but then acid production continues as the food empties out. This is why heartburn symptoms usually occur one hour after eating.

Figure 3.4   Gastroesophageal Reflux

- *Pharmacological.* The first step is to neutralize the acid that is backing up into the esophagus. Antacid preparations in liquid form work better than tablets and should be taken 1/2 to 1 hour after eating, or whenever the heartburn starts. One type of tablet forms into alkaline bubbles that sit above the liquid content of the stomach and bathe the lower esophagus. It is useful for daytime treatment. The H2 blockers also inhibit acid production, and in low or high doses can alleviate symptoms. In very severe cases of reflux, acid-inhibiting drugs called sodium-potassium pump inhibitors are prescribed. Pharmacological treatment alone, however, is not enough; reflux is a chronically occurring condition, and other measures affecting diet and lifestyle must be taken.

- *Physiological.* Because the stomach reacts to food by secreting most of its acid over 3 to 4 hours, you should eat only three meals a day, with no between-meal snacks. Do not ingest any food 3 to 4 hours before retiring at night. Sharply reduce the fat in your diet, because fat delays the emptying of the stomach. Also, a large meal with a high fat content remains in the stomach a long time, accumulates acid, and gives more opportunity for reflux. A dietary regimen of low fat, moderate protein, and high carbohydrates (preferably complex and high fiber) should be your goal. Such a diet will also relieve constipation, which exacerbates reflux. Also, avoid drinking caffeinated beverages and smoking.

- *Physical.* Eliminate all factors that increase pressure on the abdomen. This means the avoidance of tight, constricting garments—girdles, long-line brassieres, belts. If your weight is above normal or you have recently gained, weight loss, as little as 5 pounds, is recommended. To avoid nocturnal reflux, elevate the head of your bed by 4 inches or so.

■ *Surgical.* Anti-reflux surgery is reserved for those who, despite medical treatment, experience continued reflux leading to stricture, bleeding, or respiratory complications. The surgery corrects the hiatal hernia and creates a pressure zone at the end of the esophagus. If you decide to have this type of surgery, seek a highly skilled and experienced surgeon for this procedure.

Reflux in pregnancy
Reflux is a common problem in pregnancy—it is estimated that 25 percent of pregnant women have daily heartburn in the third trimester. There is obviously nothing that can be done about the pressure of the enlarging uterus on the upper abdomen, but there is some comfort in knowing that the symptoms will end at delivery. Some temporary measures can be taken to relieve the heartburn, including the spacing of meals, a low-fat diet, elevation of the head of the bed, and antacid medications that are approved by the obstetrician.

Stricture of the Esophagus
Narrowing of the esophagus is treated with dilation by special instruments or, in some cases, by surgical replacement with a section of bowel.

Cancer of the Esophagus

Practically all tumors of the esophagus are malignant. The most important risk factors are cigarette smoking and alcohol; the effects of these two factors are additive and increase the possibility of cancer. Malignant tumors of this type are twice as likely to occur in women as men. (See Fig. 3.3C)

Symptoms

Esophageal tumors usually do not produce symptoms until they have grown extensively and have seriously narrowed the diameter of the esophagus. The primary symptoms are difficulty in swallowing, weight loss, regurgitation of food, and vomiting of blood.

Diagnosis

A barium X-ray will reveal the form and the extent of the tumor, and endoscopy (esophagoscopy) can be done to take a biopsy and confirm the diagnosis. A CT scan may also be performed to determine the degree of the spread of the tumor.

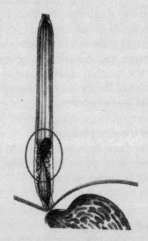

Figure 3.3C   Esophageal Cancer
This tumor grows into the esophagus and obstructs the passage of food. Dysphagia to solid food occurs first. Endoscopy with biopsy will confirm the diagnosis.

Treatment

Unfortunately, once they are discovered, very few of these tumors are amenable to surgery. If the tumor is confined to the wall of the esophagus, and has not spread beyond that organ, surgery may be successful. In other cases, radiation and chemotherapy can shrink the tumor and relieve symptoms but do not cure the tumor.

Motility Disorders

Motility disorders of the esophagus account for some cases of difficulty in swallowing: the muscles of the esophagus propel food from top to bottom in a smooth wave. The sphincter at the bottom opens as the muscular wave reaches that point, and the food is dropped into the stomach. This normal pattern is disrupted in the case of the following disorders:

- *Achalasia.* Because of a nerve dysfunction, the lower sphincter does not open properly to allow food into the stomach and the esophageal wave becomes weak. The most common symptoms are chest pain, retention of food in the esophagus, and regurgitation of recently consumed food. Diagnosis is made by means of a chest X-ray and barium esophagram, which will show the esophagus narrowing to a sharp point. Treatment consists of opening the tight sphincter either by balloon dilation or by surgery. (See Fig. 3.3D)

- *Scleroderma.* A collagen disease, scleroderma affects multiple organs and is more common in women. In close to 80 percent of scleroderma sufferers, the muscles in the lower two-thirds of the esophagus become thin and nonfunctional, and the lower sphincter becomes weak. As a result, these people suffer the symptoms and complica-

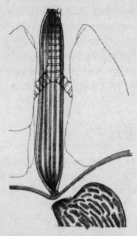

Figure 3.3D Achalasia
The lower esophageal sphincter does not relax when food is propelled down the esophagus. There is a sharply narrowed area at the end of the esophagus. Above, the esophagus is stretched and dilated.

tions of acid reflux, esophageal stricture, and changes in the lining of the esophagus. Treatment usually consists of prescribed acid-reducing medications and other anti-reflux measures and, if necessary, dilation of the esophagus to relieve stricture.

■ *Spastic disorders.* Intermittent chest pain and swallowing difficulties can be the result of diffuse esophageal spasm and other types of motility disorders. These problems are related to poorly coordinated, high-pressure esophageal contractions and a heightened sensitivity to physical and chemical stimuli within the esophagus itself. Sometimes the symptoms can be triggered by stress. It is important to eliminate any chance of the heart being the cause of the chest pain. Diagnosis can be made by barium esophagrams and manometry studies—a method of testing the motor activity of the esophagus. Treatment consists of prescribing anti-reflux measures, antidepressant medications in low doses as analgesics, smooth muscle relaxants, and, rarely, calcium channel blockers. (See Fig. 3.3E)

GI Procedures

Gastroenterologists can perform a number of specialized procedures that help to diagnose and treat condi-

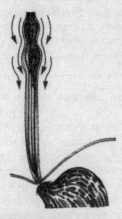

Figure 3.3E Esophageal Spasm
Uncoordinated contractions of the esophagus can result in severe chest pain, often difficult to distinguish from cardiac pain. Coronary heart disease has to be considered and eliminated in postmenopausal women or those with high risk factors. Special studies, called manometry, can detect the abnormal esophageal contractions, which can be treated by a variety of medications.

WHEN YOU HICCUP

For the most part, hiccups are a harmless annoyance. These involuntary "hics" occur when your diaphragm contracts repeatedly. As we all know, hiccups are liable to occur after a heavy meal or after drinking an excessive amount of alcohol. There are many popular remedies to get rid of an ordinary case of hiccups, including the quick downing of a glass of water while holding your breath, and breathing in and out into a paper bag. These methods may work, or the hiccups may stop on their own.

When hiccups persist for several hours or longer, see your doctor. The problem may be an irritation of the vagus nerve, which runs from the brain into your gastrointestinal system. There are also other causes of persistent hiccups, including gastritis, inflammation of the lining of the heart, and diseases of the lungs, and kidneys.

tions of the gastrointestinal system. For years X-rays, using barium as a contrast agent, were the only method for getting information about the shape and condition of the structures of the gastrointestinal tract. The upper GI series examines the esophagus, the stomach, and the duodenum. The small bowel series consists of pictures taken several hours after the GI series and shows the jejunum and the ileum. The barium enema examines the colon by introducing barium, and usually air, through the rectum, filling the colon and bringing out features of its structure. Learning to do these types of X-rays was formerly part of gastroenterology training. Now these procedures are done primarily by radiologists.

Endoscopic procedures examine the inside lining of the GI tract by use of a lighted tube. Before 1970 these tubes were rigid. Some were used to perform anoscopy, examination of the anal canal, or proctoscopy (or proctosigmoidoscopy), examination of the rectum and the lowest part of the sigmoid colon. Other rigid scopes were used to examine the esophagus and the upper part of the stomach, but they took considerable skill to use and were not for routine diagnosis. Around 1970, flexible fiber-optic scopes became available. Fiber-optic technology consisted of using extremely thin glass rods bundled together. These bundles could transmit light and images, and could be bent to go around angles in the GI tract. The first scopes were made for the stomach, then scopes to examine the colon were made. Standard procedures using these scopes have been developed.

Esophagogastroduodenoscopy, or EGD, refers to the examination of the esophagus, the stomach, and the duodenum. It is also called upper GI endoscopy. Examination of the colon is called colonoscopy. In addition to examining the walls of these structures, samples of tissue (biopsies) can be taken and therapy, like cauterizing blood vessels, can be administered. The procedures are done in a specially equipped suite in a hospital or a doctor's office. For EGD, fasting is required. A local anesthetic is given to numb the back of the throat, and a sedative may be administered. For colonoscopy, a 2-day cleansing procedure is done to empty the colon. A mild sedative may be given. The time required for these procedures depends on whether biopsies are taken or therapy, like cautery of bleeding vessels, is performed.

Endoscopic retrograde cholangiopancreatography (ERCP) combines endoscopy with radiography to show the pattern of ducts coming from the liver and the pancreas. It is particularly useful in showing stones or changes in the duct systems caused by tumors or inflammations. In operative ERCP, stones can be removed, or tubes placed to bypass segments of ducts blocked by tumor.

It is beyond the scope of this chapter to describe in detail all the specialized procedures used for the GI tract. Some of them are done only in research centers and are not generally available. Reference is made to some specialized procedures in the discussions of various conditions.

DISORDERS OF THE STOMACH

A pear-shaped, muscular organ, the stomach lies mostly on the left-hand side below the ribs. It receives food from the esophagus and produces the churning action that mixes the food with digestive enzymes and acid, reducing it to a thin liquid.

From time to time, the stomach fails to work properly and you may experience indigestion. The discomfort is usually self-limiting and passes quickly. If indigestion is persistent, however, it may be a sign of a more serious illness and merits consulting a doctor for a diagnosis. (See Fig. 3.5)

Gastritis

Gastritis is a term used to describe inflammation or damage to the stomach lining. (Gastritis is not to be confused with gastroenteritis, which is a short-lived illness, usually caused by a virus. Called intestinal flu, it is characterized by vomiting, diarrhea, abdominal cramps, and fever.) The two most common types of gastritis are atrophic gastritis and erosive, or hemorrhagic, gastritis. *Atrophic* gastritis is characterized by the loss of the stomach cells that are responsible for manufacturing acid, pepsin, and intrinsic factor, which is a complex protein necessary for the absorption of vitamin B12. This

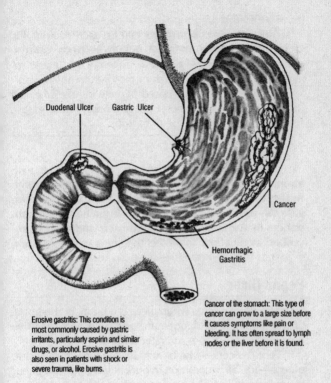

Duodenal Ulcer   Gastric Ulcer

Cancer

Hemorrhagic
Gastritis

Erosive gastritis: This condition is
most commonly caused by gastric
irritants, particularly aspirin and similar
drugs, or alcohol. Erosive gastritis is
also seen in patients with shock or
severe trauma, like burns.

Cancer of the stomach: This type of
cancer can grow to a large size before
it causes symptoms like pain or
bleeding. It has often spread to lymph
nodes or the liver before it is found.

Figure 3.5   Disorders of the Stomach

condition occurs in older people or those suffering from
a long-term infection with *Helicobacter pylori. Erosive*
gastritis occurs when shallow ulcers or sores develop on
the upper layer of the stomach lining, usually because of
the excessive ingestion of a stomach irritant such as
aspirin or alcohol. It can occur in critically ill patients
because of poor blood supply to the stomach.

Symptoms

Atrophic gastritis produces no symptoms. Bleeding is the most common symptom of hemmorhagic gastritis.

Diagnosis

Gastritis is best diagnosed by viewing the stomach interior through an endoscope. A biopsy of the gastric tissue determines the type of gastritis.

Treatment

If a B12 deficiency develops, as may occur with atrophic gastritis, you will need lifelong treatment with monthly vitamin B12 injections. In the case of erosive gastritis, you will have to discontinue the use of any substances that are irritating to the stomach, and may be prescribed medications to protect the lining of the stomach.

Peptic Ulcer

A peptic ulcer occurs when there is a break in the lining of the stomach or duodenum, and acid and digestive enzymes cause a sore or crater to form.

Peptic ulcers—which include duodenal and gastric ulcers—are fairly common in our society, and can occur at any time of life. The precise cause is still open to question. Contrary to popular belief, ulcers are not confined to high-powered executives or to people under a lot of stress. There is some proof, however, that the disposition to form ulcers is inherited.

The digestive enzyme pepsin and stomach acids are essential for ulcer formation. Caffeine, for example, stimulates pepsin and acid secretion. Alcohol, aspirin, and nonsteroidal anti-inflammatory drugs (NSAIDs) can disrupt the lining of the digestive tract. Cigarette smoking is associated with ulcer formation, although the mechanism is unknown. Recent studies have discovered that a significant number of peptic ulcer patients have infection of the stomach lining with the bacterium *Helicobacter pylori*.

Symptoms

A burning, gnawing pain in the upper middle abdomen is the most common symptom of a peptic ulcer. The area surrounding the ulcer can become irritated and cause the underlying muscles to develop spasms; the nerve endings are then activated, causing pain. It usually occurs on an empty stomach, before meals, or in the middle of the night. You may also experience bloating, nausea, and vomiting.

In some cases, a blood vessel can erode and cause bleeding. The bleeding may be detected only by a study of the stool, or massive bleeding can occur, causing the vomiting of blood. Vomited blood may appear as black particles, called coffee grounds. Alternatively, the blood may pass through the intestinal tract, resulting in a tarry stool. Weakness and dizziness may accompany the bleeding. This is an emergency, and medical help should be sought as soon as possible.

Diagnosis

Because peptic ulcer can be a chronic condition, it is most helpful to have a definitive diagnosis at the outset. If you are experiencing the typical symptoms of an ulcer, your physician will start you on a therapeutic trial of antacid therapy immediately, before any tests are performed. (A dramatic response to antacids strongly favors the presence of an ulcer.) She or he will then make arrangements for an X-ray test called an upper gastrointestinal series (GI series). The GI series will show ulcers that have penetrated the muscular wall of the stomach or duodenum, but will not detect shallow ulcers. Endoscopy detects both shallow and deep ulcers, and a culture and biopsy can detect the presence of *Helico-*

bacter bacterium. Evidence of *Helicobacter* infection can also be found by a blood antibody test or a breath test.

In cases of massive bleeding, the diagnosis must be made immediately. In this situation, an upper endoscopy can locate the ulcer. Active bleeding can be controlled by cautery. If this does not stop the bleeding, abdominal surgery is necessary.

Treatment

Because peptic ulcers can recur and cause serious complications, it is important to lessen any chances of a return of the condition. There is no special diet for ulcers. At one time, the typical ulcer diet consisted of bland foods, with heavy emphasis on milk and milk products, but this is no longer considered important or particularly effective. However, it *is* recommended that you eliminate alcohol and caffeine from your diet, avoid the use of aspirin and certain other drugs, and stop smoking. The mainstay of treatment is the removal of acid from the stomach. This is done by means of antacids, which neutralize stomach acid, or H2 blockers, which keep the stomach cells from making acid, or a combination of both. If the *Helicobacter* bacterium is present, antibiotics are added. Eliminating *Helicobacter* from the stomach markedly decreases the likelihood that the ulcer will recur.

Once your ulcer has healed, your doctor may advise you to continue taking a smaller dose of an H2 blocker on a regular basis, to eliminate any chance of the ulcer recurring. Duodenal ulcers are assumed to be healed in about eight weeks if the pain disappears. Healing of a gastric ulcer has to be confirmed by X-ray or endoscopy, to ensure that a gastric cancer is not responsible for the appearance of the ulcer. Surgery is seldom required, unless the ulcer does not heal with medication, or there are complications like bleeding or obstruction.

THE SYMPTOMS OF INDIGESTION

We're all familiar with the symptoms of indigestion: discomfort or a feeling of fullness in the upper abdomen, nausea, heartburn, bloating, and a tendency to belch. Indigestion is caused by eating certain foods, too much alcohol, stress, eating too fast, or has no discernible cause.

Persistent indigestion can be a symptom of a major underlying disease, such as peptic ulcer, gastritis, gallbladder disease, or cancer. If you suffer from chronic abdominal discomfort, seek medical help. Once your doctor has established the pattern of your symptoms—when they occur, their intensity, and their duration—he or she may have to run tests to rule out any serious disorder or disease that may be causing the problem. These tests include barium X-ray studies, ultrasound, and CT scans.

It may happen that no reason is found for your abdominal discomfort. In that case, the doctor may prescribe antacids or an acid-reducing medication and advise certain modifications in your diet and lifestyle. You may be asked to stop drinking or smoking, for example, or to avoid stressful situations that may exacerbate your condition. If a specific cause for your discomfort is found—such as gastritis or an ulcer—your physician can recommend the appropriate treatment.

Stomach Tumors

As with tumors of the esophagus, the majority of stomach tumors are malignant. Fortunately, for unknown reasons, this type of tumor is decreasing in incidence in the United States. Diet may play a role in the formation of a gastric tumor, but there is no conclusive proof of this.

Symptoms

Because the stomach is a large and flexible organ, tumors arising from the stomach lining grow significantly and may spread to the lymph nodes and liver before they are discovered. The most frequent symptoms are upper abdominal pain, blood in the stools, weight loss, and an iron deficiency anemia resulting from slow blood loss. If the tumor blocks the esophagus or the pylorus (the outlet of the stomach), it may be found at an earlier stage, and thus have a better chance of a surgical cure.

Diagnosis

Because the symptoms of a gastric tumor are similar to those of a peptic ulcer, there is no one symptom that indicates cancer of the stomach. Again, a barium X-ray or an endoscopic examination can determine the location of the problem, and a biopsy can identify a possible cancer. CT scans may be necessary to ascertain if the disease has spread to adjoining organs.

Treatment

If the tumor is malignant, surgery is the only treatment that offers any chance of a cure, depending on the spread of the disease. Chemotherapy and radiation may shrink the tumor and provide temporary improvement, but no curative regimen has been developed to date. Even when surgery cannot cure the condition, it still may be recommended to remove blockages, arrest bleeding, or help alleviate pain.

DISORDERS OF THE INTESTINES

After food has been broken down by stomach acid and enzymes, it passes slowly into the small intestine, which consists of the duodenum, the jejunum, and the ileum. Here the nutrients are absorbed into the bloodstream through the lining of the small intestine. Undigested food, water, and other intestinal waste pass into the large intestine—consisting of the colon and the rectum—where they are solidified and prepared for excretion.

The intestines are where the major part of digestion takes place: nutrients are absorbed into the bloodstream for distribution throughout the body, water and salt are reabsorbed, and wastes are eliminated. Many of the disorders afflicting this part of the digestive system involve inflammation from infections, malabsorption, and intestinal obstructions.

Infections of the Intestinal Tract

Intestinal infections—whether viral, bacterial, or parasitic—are extremely common. Babies as well as adults get them, and travelers to other counties are especially susceptible. The infectious agents are spread mainly by food or water contaminated by human waste. *Gastroenteritis* disturbs the function of the stomach and the small intestine; *dysentery* generally refers to severe infections of the large intestine.

- *Viral gastroenteritis.* This type of infection usually begins with fever and vomiting followed by diarrhea. A number of different viruses can cause this illness, which is easily transmitted by person-to-person contact. The actual infection lasts only a few days, but symptoms, particularly diarrhea, can be prolonged by a too hasty resumption of the normal diet.

- *Bacterial gastroenteritis.* A staphylococcal intestinal infection is caused by a toxin produced by bacteria in food that is allowed to sit too long at room temperature. Vomiting begins within a few hours after eating the food, followed by diarrhea. The symptoms usually vanish by the next day. *Salmonella* is a bacterium that can be present in raw eggs or incompletely cooked chicken. *Shigella* and *Campylobacter* organisms primarily affect the colon and can cause blood to appear in the stool. (Typhoid fever, which is caused by *Salmonella,* is rare in the United States, but travelers to developing countries who plan to spend time in rural areas are encouraged to take a course of typhoid immunization for protection.) These three organisms can be cultured from the stool and treated with antibiotics.

- *Parasitic infections.* These infections, which include giardiasis and amebiasis, are common and cause a variety of digestive illnesses. They are usually transmitted to travelers by close contact or by a contaminated water supply. Again, the agent is usually identified by testing the stool. They are treated with antiparasitic medication.

Treatment of infectious diarrhea

When diarrhea occurs, the enterocytes, or cells lining the small intestine, replace themselves at a rapid rate. These cells are immature and are not capable of specialized digestive and absorptive functions. Eating foods that are simple to digest and then gradually adding more complex foods will provide an easier transition back to a normal diet. For example:

- *Acute phase*—plenty of fluids: tea, clear soup. Solid food should be saltine crackers, rice, dry toast.

- *Next few days*—plain meat, no fat. Other food could include banana, cooked fruits and vegetables.

As the days progress, slowly reintroduce raw fruits and vegetables, fats, and dairy products.

How to avoid traveler's diarrhea

Whether called turista or Montezuma's revenge, traveler's diarrhea (TD) can quickly put a damper on a vacation. Generally, the highest-risk destinations are the developing nations of Latin America, Africa, the Middle East, and Asia. Although the infection can be caused by a virus, bacterium, or parasite, the most common culprit is the *E. coli* bacterium, which releases a toxin that causes the intestines to pour out large amounts of secretions, especially fluids.

To prevent traveler's diarrhea, make sure to do the following:

- Drink only bottled water or beverages. Do not use ice in drinks unless it has been made from disinfected water.

- Peel raw fruits and vegetables before eating them. Do not eat raw meat or raw seafood.

- Never eat street-vendor food. Eat cooked food as soon after it is cooked as possible.

- Wash your hands even more than usual, particularly before meals and before handling food.

Traveler's diarrhea is annoying and disruptive, and every victim wants relief from cramping and the "runs."

Popular remedies include a kaolin-pectin preparation (Kaopectate) and bismuth (Pepto-Bismol), which contains an anti-inflammatory agent, bismuth subsalicylate. Diphenoxylate (Lomotil) and loperamide (Imodium) slow intestinal transit. These drugs can provide temporary relief, but should not be used if the diarrhea continues for more than a few days. (It's best not to treat mild diarrhea for the first few hours; it may be the body's way of purging itself of an intestinal infection.) Severe diarrhea, which produces dehydration, fever, and blood in the stool, requires the attention of a doctor.

If you suffer from acute diarrhea, it is vital that you replace lost fluids to avoid dehydration. Drink beverages containing sugar, consomme, and bottled water.

Malabsorption Disorders

Many different types of diseases and conditions can interfere with the normal digestive or absorptive mechanisms of the small intestine. This is called malabsorption. Vital nutrients, instead of entering the bloodstream, are eliminated in the stool. This inability to absorb vitamins can lead to anemia (loss of vitamin B12 or folate), changes in the skin (loss of vitamin A), weakening of the bones (loss of vitamin D), and disruption of normal blood clotting (loss of vitamin K).

Symptoms
The signs of malabsorption include a general feeling of weakness, weight loss, diarrhea, abdominal cramps, excess gas, bloating, and foul-smelling stools that float in the toilet bowl.

Diagnosis
The most important diagnostic test is the fecal fat test; more than 5 grams of fat eliminated in the stool over a 24-hour period indicates a significant malabsorption

problem. A series of other tests, including blood tests, X-rays, and function tests, can track down the cause.

Lactose intolerance

Lactose is a sugar found in milk and other fresh dairy products. A double sugar, lactose must be split into its two components before being absorbed. Lactase, the enzyme that splits this sugar, is located on the edges of the mature small intestinal cells. Although most people are able to digest milk in infancy, those descended from populations that traditionally did not eat a dairy-based diet—African, Asian, Mediterranean, and Near Eastern peoples—lose their ability to digest milk, usually because the amount of lactase in their intestinal cells decreases with age.

When lactose is not split and absorbed in the upper part of the small intestine, it moves on down the gastrointestinal tract and is split by the bacteria in the lower small bowel and the colon. The sugars are broken down into gases and irritating acids, which cause bloating, loose stools, cramps, and abdominal gas. The symptoms occur anywhere from 2 to 6 hours after consuming lactose. Diagnosis is confirmed by a lactose tolerance test. Treatment consists of avoiding fresh milk and foods made from milk, such as ice cream. If you want or need to drink milk, you can treat it with lactase; when you eat lactose-rich foods, you can take a lactase tablet. (Treated milk can be made into other foods.) Because the lactose in aged cheeses and yogurt has been already split by the culturing organisms, these products can be eaten without difficulty.

Celiac (nontropical) sprue

An inherited disorder, celiac disease is characterized by an intolerance to gluten, a protein found in certain grains, including wheat, oats, rye, and barley. The gluten causes an inflammatory reaction in the upper small intestine that totally changes the structure of the cells and interferes with absorption of nutrients. Common symptoms are bloated stomach, foul-smelling stools, and anemia. Celiac disease usually appears in childhood; children with the disorder lose weight and fail to grow. The main treatment is the elimination from the diet of foods containing gluten. Because gluten is a common ingredient of many processed foods, it is necessary to examine labels very carefully to make sure it is not in a particular item. People suffering from celiac disease may profit from the advice of a nutritionist, to make sure they are consuming an adequate, healthy diet.

Chronic pancreatitis
Conditions of the pancreas can lead to malabsorption. (See section on pancreas in this chapter.)

Acute Appendicitis

The appendix is a worm-shaped blind pouch of varying size that extends off the cecum, the first segment of the colon. It is located in the right lower abdomen. The appendix has some digestive function in some mammalian species, but has no known function or importance in humans except occasionally to cause trouble. Appendicitis occurs when a hard piece of stool blocks the opening of the appendix, causing swelling, inflammation, and infection. The appendix can then rupture, and a localized infection, called an abscess, can form. Or a more generalized infection can spread over the surface of adjacent organs, causing peritonitis. Both of these events are medical emergencies and require immediate surgery. (See Fig. 3.6)

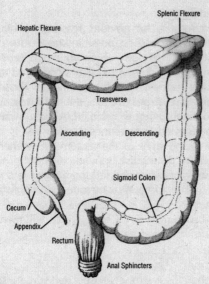

Figure 3.6   The Colon
The colon (large intestine) is distributed in a U-shape in the abdomen. Its main sections are the ascending, transverse, descending and sigmoid portions, ending in the rectum. Endoscopic diagnostic procedures on the colon are described according to how many sections of the colon are seen. Colonoscopy means that the scope was passed from the rectum all the way around to the cecum. Flexible sigmoidoscopy, the screening procedure, attempts to see the rectum, the sigmoid, and the descending colon, if possible. Cancers and polyps are more common on the left side. Proctoscopy, with a rigid instrument, covers the rectum and the beginning of the sigmoid.

Symptoms

Appendicitis usually begins with a vague pain in the middle of the abdomen. The pain becomes sharper as it localizes to the right lower abdomen. Other symptoms are loss of appetite, nausea and vomiting, and constipation.

Diagnosis

It is important, for obvious reasons, to diagnose appendicitis at the earliest possible stage. Your doctor will question you carefully about your symptoms, and will palpate your abdomen to elicit a "rebound tenderness" over the area where the appendix lies. The tenderness signifies that the peritoneum, the sensitive covering of the abdominal lining, is inflamed. A rectal exam will also be performed; sometimes tenderness is found above and to the right of the rectum. In women it is often difficult to distinguish appendicitis from problems affecting the right ovary and fallopian tube, so a pelvic exam is advisable. Other tests include a white blood cell count—when elevated, it can signal a bacterial infection—and a sonogram or CT scan, which will reveal the appendix and surrounding organs.

Treatment

If appendicitis is strongly suspected, surgery should be done immediately. The appendix is removed and the base tied off. Laparoscopic surgery is a recent development that can be used to treat cases of uncomplicated appendicitis.

Inflammatory Bowel Disease

Inflammatory bowel disease (IBD) is a general term that applies to two diseases of unknown cause that involve the intestines: Crohn's disease and ulcerative colitis. *Crohn's disease*—also called ileitis, regional enteritis, or Crohn's colitis—is a chronic inflammation of both small and large intestines. *Ulcerative colitis* is a chronic condition characterized by ulcers and abscesses of the large intestine only. Although these diseases can strike at any time in life, the peak time of onset is about age 20. Both conditions tend to run in some families.

Symptoms

Chronic diarrhea, abdominal cramps, rectal bleeding, fatigue, low-grade fever, and weight loss are common symptoms of both Crohn's disease and ulcerative colitis.

MALABSORPTION AS A RESULT OF WEIGHT-LOSS SURGERY

A few severely obese people, desperate to lose weight, choose to undergo a jejunal-ileal bypass operation, which excludes long portions of the nutrient-absorbing surfaces of the small intestine. This operation has been associated with numerous nutritional deficiencies and complications, including gallstones, kidney stones, and liver disease. One unfortunate result of the surgery is that undigested fat moves down the intestinal tract, causing the typical symptoms of malabsorption: bloating, diarrhea, and foul-smelling gas and stools.

Because of these problems, other types of weight-loss surgical procedures are now favored over the intestinal bypass operation. One such operation is a gastric bypass or gastroplasty, which drastically reduces the storage capacity of the stomach. It allows only a small amount of food to be eaten at one time but leaves the absorptive organs intact. Side effects of a gastric bypass can include deficiencies in vitamin B12, folate, and iron.

Research is also being done on a lipase inhibitor, a drug that interferes with the enzyme that is necessary for the digestion and absorption of fat.

Diagnosis

Both Crohn's disease and ulcerative colitis are life-long conditions that can range from mild to life-threatening. For that reason, their management is best left in the hands of a specialist in gastroenterology. If one of these disorders is suspected, the physician will run a series of tests to establish a diagnosis. If bleeding is present, the first test is a sigmoidoscopy to examine the condition of the lining of the rectum and sigmoid colon. (See Fig. 3.7) A barium X-ray or colonoscopy, to see the entire interior of the colon, may be performed to determine the extent of the disease in the colon. An upper GI series with a small bowel follow-through (barium X-rays) determines whether there is involvement of the small bowel.

Treatment

A mild case of Crohn's disease may require no treatment except anti-diarrheal medication. If the problem is more acute, anti-inflammatory medications, such as sulfasalazine or prednisone, are used. Sometimes immunosuppressant drugs are prescribed to inhibit the inflammatory reaction. Surgery is done to remove obstructions. Efforts are made to avoid surgery because the condition tends to recur.

Treatment of ulcerative colitis includes medications to control inflammation and diarrhea. A few patients may not improve and develop severe disease of the entire colon, requiring surgery to remove the diseased colon and rectum. Removing all colon tissue is curative in ulcerative colitis but results in an ileostomy—the attachment of the end of the ileum to the abdominal wall. Waste material drains into a bag attached to the abdomen. A new procedure called an ileoanal anastomosis is now being performed. This operation leaves intact the anus and its sphincter muscles, which are then attached to the small intestine, allowing waste matter to exit normally.

Active research on the causes and therapy of both these serious disorders is ongoing. To find out more about inflammatory bowel disease, get in touch with The Crohn's & Colitis Foundation of America, 386 Park Avenue South, 17th floor, New York, NY 10016-8804. This organization funds research and provides educational materials and support networks for patients and families.

Irritable Bowel Syndrome

This syndrome has several names: spastic colon, spastic colitis, mucus colitis, or functional bowel disease. *Colitis* is actually an inaccurate term, because no infection or inflammation is present. In fact, the diagnosis is based on the absence of evidence of other intestinal disorders. Because the symptoms are so variable, many people suffer with this problem for years before seeking help. Irritable bowel syndrome usually starts in the teen years or young adulthood. Women are more affected than men. (See Fig. 3.7)

Symptoms

The symptoms seem to be the result of two disorders of intestinal function: abnormal motility (impaired contractions of the intestine) and increased sensitivity to bowel distention. Constipation, diarrhea, alternating constipation and diarrhea, cramping, gas, and bloating are all common symptoms. Typically, the symptoms occur after a meal and are often relieved by a bowel movement. Constipation is a common complaint, and many people suffering from this disorder use laxatives excessively, which exacerbates the condition. Stress and depression appear to play a role in many patients.

Diagnosis

Don't suffer in silence if you experience the chronic symptoms of irritable bowel syndrome. See your physician to make sure there is no underlying disease causing the problem. A physical exam can reveal the presence of intestinal gas and variable areas of tenderness in the abdomen. Other tests, including standard blood tests, sigmoidoscopy, and possibly barium enema or colonoscopy, confirm the diagnosis by revealing no other condition. An anoscopy may find complications of constipation—hemorrhoids or fissures.

Treatment

Increasing the fiber content of the diet can improve the motor function of the bowel and result in a formed, regular stool. Adequate amounts of fiber must be con-

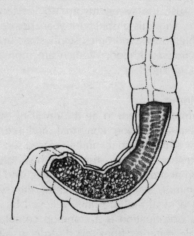

Figure 3.7 Inflammatory Bowel Disease
A segment of colon, showing colitis. The normal folds are disrupted by multiple ulcers and swollen inflamed tissue called "pseudopolyps." This tissue can bleed and secrete excessive mucus, resulting in what has been named the "currant jelly" stool.

sumed daily: three to five servings of fruit and four to five servings of vegetables, and whole-grain breads and cereals, for a total of 20 grams of fiber. Use bulk laxatives when there is a problem getting adequate fibrous food, as can happen when traveling. Occasionally a low dose of antidepressants, which can alter the perception of pain signals from the bowel, is helpful. Biofeedback and psychological counseling can also aid in relieving stress.

Diverticular Disease

A diverticulum is a pouch that develops in the colon and protrudes through its wall. (In an X-ray, diverticula look like marbles sitting on the outside of the colon.) The pouches are caused by high-pressure pockets that occur when the colon is relatively empty—the colon lining is forced out through the weak spots where the blood vessels penetrate the intestinal muscle. *Diverticulosis* is the term used to describe the state of having diverticula in the colon. *Diverticulitis* refers to an inflammatory condition of the pouch or pouches. (See Fig. 3.8)

The disease is a condition of advancing years: 10 percent of 50-year-olds have diverticulosis, and 50 percent of 90-year-olds suffer from it. The main cause seems to be our low-fiber diet, which forces the colon to generate high pressures to move the food along, leading to a collapse at certain parts of the colon wall. Once the pouches develop, they remain a lifelong threat.

Symptoms

Many people with diverticulosis have no symptoms and are not aware that they have the condition. Others suffer from various symptoms, including abdominal pain (usually on the left side), fever, nausea, and sometimes rectal bleeding.

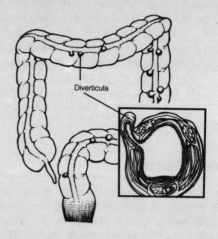

Figure 3.8 Diverticulosis
Diverticula are small pouches of colon lining that protrude through the muscular wall of the colon. They are caused by high pressure on potentially weak areas where the blood vessels penetrate the wall. They are more common on the left side of the colon than on the right. These pouches can become inflamed and infected, "diverticulitis," causing pain and fever. Occasionally they can perforate and cause a diverticular abscess.

Diagnosis

A case of diverticulosis may be noticed only incidentally, when X-rays or a colonoscopy is being performed for other reasons. If you do suffer from a severe pain in your lower left abdomen, a diverticulum may have become inflamed or infected as a result of food and bacteria lodging in it. If neglected, diverticulitis can result in infection and perforation with abscess formation, which requires immediate medical attention. The diagnosis is usually made by the clinical examination. Ultrasound or CT scanning can locate an abscess that has formed.

Treatment

Diverticulosis symptoms of pain in the lower abdomen without a sign of infection are best treated with a high-fiber diet to improve muscular function and to lower colon pressures. Severe pain with signs of infection—fever, elevated white blood cell count—usually means that the diverticulum has become obstructed

---

TYPES OF LAXATIVES

There are a number of different kinds of medications that stimulate defecation:

- *Bulk laxatives*—increase the amount of insoluble fiber and stimulate more effective muscular activity of the intestines.
- *Saline laxatives*—contain unabsorbable compounds, like magnesium oxide, that keep water in the intestine and make the stool more liquid.
- *Stool softeners*—make the stool easier to pass.
- *Stimulant laxatives*—cause increased activity of the colon muscles.
- *Irritant laxatives* (castor oil)—paralyze the small intestine's absorptive mechanism, resulting in a large increase of fluid in the intestine.

Laxatives can be helpful when you have an occasional bout of constipation. However, it's rare for anyone to need laxatives on a daily basis; excessive use of laxatives can actually lead to weakness of the colon muscles, contributing to the problem they are meant to prevent: constipation. Instead of relying on laxatives, try making these changes in your lifestyle:

- Drink lots of fluids, including six to eight glasses of water a day.
- Alter your diet to include a lot more fiber. You can do this by eating more fruits and vegetables on a daily basis.
- Exercise regularly.
- When nature calls, do not suppress the urge to move your bowels. If at all possible, go to the bathroom.
- Do not use enemas on a regular basis. They interfere with the natural process of defecation.
- If you must use a laxative, use a bulk laxative.

and infected; in some cases there can be rupture with abscess formation. Hospitalization with intravenous feeding, antibiotics, and possibly surgery is required to control and resolve the infection. Another diverticulosis syndrome is sudden, copious, bright red rectal bleeding that is the result of erosion of the blood vessel next to the opening of the diverticulum. This usually resolves spontaneously, without treatment.

If you experience frequent attacks of diverticulitis, it may be advisable to have the involved segment of the bowel removed surgically.

Growths in the Colon: Polyps and Tumors

Polyps are small growths on the inside lining of the intestine. The muscular action of the intestine pulls on them, sometimes creating a stalk, so polyps often resemble mushrooms. (See Fig. 3.9) There are several types of polyps found in the colon; the most common are hyperplastic and adenomatous. *Hyperplastic* polyps are not a health risk and are not associated with the development of colon cancer. *Adenomatous* polyps, on the other hand, have the potential to become cancerous. The discovery of an adenomatous polyp in the colon is a signal to perform a full colonoscopy, remove all polyps found, and continue to monitor the patient regularly thereafter.

Symptoms
Often there are no symptoms, and the polyps are found during a screening sigmoidoscopy or a diagnostic markup for blood in the stool. Rarely, polyps may cause visible blood in the stool or a change in bowel movements.

Diagnosis
The definitive diagnosis is made by microscopic examination of the polyp, or part of it, by a pathologist.

Treatment

Most polyps are removed when detected, to eliminate any chance they will become malignant later. If an adenomatous polyp is found, you should be monitored periodically for other growths in the colon.

Colorectal Cancer

Cancer of the colon and rectum is the second most common cancer (after breast cancer) in women in the United States. Women and men are affected equally. The development of colorectal cancer is thought to be related to our high-fat, low-fiber diet as well as to specific

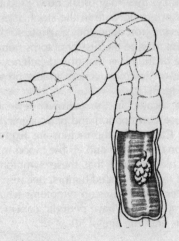

Figure 3.9   Colon Polyp
A polyp begins as a heaped-up area of tissue. As it grows, the intestinal motion pulls it, creating a stalk. Most polyps are benign (not cancerous), but some types of polyps may develop into cancer. If an adenomatous or villous polyp is discovered on screening, the entire colon should be looked at (colonoscopy) and all polyps removed.

genetic factors. The incidence of colon cancer increases sharply in those over 50, so periodic screening for this type of tumor should begin at that age. Standard screening consists of a physical examination by the physician—the digital rectal exam—plus a three-day test for occult blood in the stool, proctoscopy, or flexible sigmoidoscopy. Proctoscopy is a direct visual examination of the lower part of the colon, the rectum; a flexible sigmoidoscopy examines the rectum, the sigmoid colon, and sometimes the descending colon. (See Fig. 3.6)

Symptoms
Symptoms depend on the location of the cancer. Cancers formed in the large-diameter right side of the colon are bulky; they may break down and bleed, but the blood is not noticeable in the stool. These cancers can cause severe iron deficiency anemia, so that fatigue and weakness may be the first symptoms noticed. (One medical rule of thumb is that iron deficiency in a middle-aged person is colon cancer unless proven otherwise.) (See Fig. 3.10)

Cancers located in the narrower left side of the colon produce constipation and pain, signifying partial obstruction. Cancers in the rectum are likely to cause discomfort on defecation and visible blood in the stool. It must be remembered that these symptoms are all indicative of fairly advanced tumors. Because early colorectal cancer often causes no symptoms whatever, it is extremely important to have periodic cancer screening examinations after the age of 50.

Treatment
Surgery is the primary treatment of choice for colon cancer. The diseased colon is removed and the draining lymph nodes are checked for any sign of spreading cancer. Surgery for cancer in the rectum depends on how

deeply the tumor has penetrated the wall. Radiation and chemotherapy have been shown to decrease recurrence and improve the patient's chances of survival.

Anorectal Disorders

The anus is the outlet for the rectum. Anorectal disorders tend to involve inflammations, abscesses, hemorrhoids, and fissures.

Anorectal Abscess, Perianal Abscess, and Fistula

An *anorectal abscess* is usually the result of an infection of one of the anal glands. A *perianal abscess* occurs when the infection develops under the skin around the anal opening. The main complication of these infections

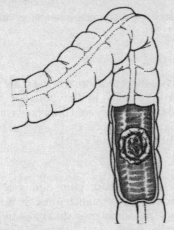

Figure 3.10 Colon Cancer
Colon cancer invades the wall of the colon and may have a flat, ulcerated appearance. Sometimes it will affect the entire circumference of the colon and produce what is called an "apple core" or "napkin ring" appearance.

is the development of a *fistula*, an abnormal connection or passageway between the anus or rectum and the perianal skin.

Symptoms
Anal abscesses cause dull to severe pain in or around the anal opening, accompanied by fever. If you have anal pain and fever, you should consult a physician immediately. A *fistula* will cause the skin around the anus to become itchy and irritated because of fluid and secretions draining from the hole.

Diagnosis
A physical exam is usually all that is necessary to diagnose anorectal abscess, perianal abscess, or fistula.

Treatment
Anal abscesses are a surgical emergency and must be drained.

Anal Fissure
An anal fissure is an ulcer that forms in the outer portion of the anal canal, usually in the posterior section, toward the backbone. Fissures are commonly caused by the passage of large, hard stools that cause splits in the skin in a weak area of the anal canal.

Symptoms
Anal fissures cause sharp pain during and after defecation, especially if the sphincter muscle is irritated and goes into spasm. Sometimes streaks of bright red blood appear on the stool.

Diagnosis
The fissure can usually be seen by the physician upon examination, although anoscopy may be per-

formed to confirm the finding. Stool softeners and bulking agents can promote easier passage of the stool. A sitz bath—sitting in a tub of hot water for 20 minutes—can relax the perianal muscles and increase the blood supply to the tissue, thus promoting healing. A chronic fissure that resists healing by conservative means can be treated surgically. A colorectal surgeon or a general surgeon with extensive experience in proctology is the specialist to perform this procedure.

Hemorrhoids

Three spongy cushions, containing a rich supply of veins, lie under the lining of the anal canal. The wear and tear of elimination—and chronic constipation—can stretch these tissues and cause the veins inside them to enlarge and protrude through the canal, causing the formation of hemorrhoids, or "piles." At times, clots can form in the veins and ulcers can form, resulting in severe pain and bleeding. Pregnancy is a high-risk time for the development of hemorrhoids, especially in the third trimester. (See Fig. 3.11)

Symptoms

The main symptoms of hemorrhoids are feelings of pain and pressure in the anal canal, usually after a hard bowel movement, an episode of diarrhea, or lifting a heavy object. A grapelike lump may be present at the anal opening. You may also notice bright red blood on the toilet paper or on the stool itself, tenderness, and a protrusion of soft tissue at the anal opening. Rectal bleeding, whether you think it is from hemorrhoids or not, should be brought to medical attention and investigated.

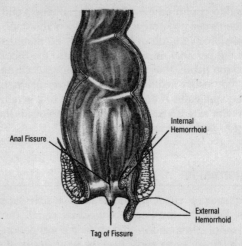

Figure 3.11 Conditions of the Anorectum
Hemorrhoids: Internal hemorrhoids originate from the upper part of the anal canal and are generally contained within it. External hemorrhoids originate from a lower plexus of vessels and may result in lumps protruding from the anus.

Diagnosis
The hemorrhoid can usually be seen or felt during the examination by your physician. The area will be examined by an anoscope or proctoscope to confirm the finding.

Treatment
Hemorrhoids are not a disease, merely a symptom of wear and tear. The best treatment, then, is to alter the factors that lead to their formation. Treatment of acute hemorrhoids is the same as for an anal fissure—softening the stool, sitz baths, and topical anal lubricants. Most cases of hemorrhoids can be relieved by

these simple measures. There are surgical procedures that can provide relief, but they are not usually necessary.

Complications of hemorrhoids

When hemorrhoids heal, they may leave a tag of redundant tissue. When numerous tags form, the anal cushions may become less competent, allowing a seepage of irritating secretions and causing a condition called pruritis ani. Rarely, hemorrhoids can be source of significant blood loss, causing anemia. Both of these conditions can benefit from surgery. As with anal fissures, only an experienced surgeon should be chosen to perform this procedure. The most important component of treatment, however, is lifelong changes in diet, weight loss, and other measures to ease the passage of stools and decrease pressure on the anal cushions.

Anal Itching

Pruritis ani, or itching around the anal opening, is a common condition that should be promptly investigated and treated. Scratching, wiping, washing, and the use of over-the-counter remedies can make this condition worse and harder to treat.

Symptoms

In rare instances, the symptom of itching can be due to pinworm, a parasite that is usually brought home by a child from school or day care and spread through the family. More commonly, the symptom is from stool left behind because of incomplete wiping, multiple hemorrhoid tags (see above), or the seepage of irritating secretions from fistulas or a weakened sphincter. Constant moisture in the area can also make the skin vulnerable to fungal infection that causes itching. In some cases,

FECAL INCONTINENCE

In most instances, our anal sphincter mechanisms are able to control the excretion of gas and liquid or solid feces. Occasionally, even in healthy people, this mechanism can be overwhelmed, usually by a severe case of diarrhea and the absence of a readily accessible toilet. Such occurrences are embarrassing but should not be a cause for alarm. If they continue, however, consult a doctor. The most common causes are specific anal conditions, complications of anal or rectal surgery, and obstetrical injury.

Your doctor will give you a thorough physical examination, checking for normal nerve function, anatomical deformities, and the strength of the anal sphincter muscles. If necessary, you can take more sophisticated tests that measure pressure in the rectum and anus. Treatment varies according to the condition. You may profit from changes in diet and medications to make the stool solid, and exercises that increase the strength of the external anal sphincter can also be helpful. Injuries from prior surgery and obstetrical trauma can be repaired by a colorectal specialist.

Because fecal incontinence can result from previous surgery and similar trauma, it is important to remember that surgery should never be done for hemorrhoids, fissures, or fistulas unless it is patently necessary, and then only by a surgeon with extensive experience in the specialty. In childbirth, the posterolateral episiotomy incision is much safer than the direct posterior episiotomy, which can extend through the anal sphincter from the extreme pressure of the baby's head or during forceps delivery.

too vigorous wiping and cleaning of the anal area can lead to irritation and itching.

Diagnosis
Your physician will look for pinworm, fistula, hemorrhoids, and skin changes, and check the strength of the anal sphincter.

Treatment
Any identified problems should be treated, but often no such problems are present. If that is the case, then a concerted effort must be made to stop the scratching, which damages the skin and stimulates more itching. Other suggestions:

- Discontinue all over-the-counter anti-itch medications, since some ingredients may cause a local dermatitis.
- After using the toilet, wipe yourself with water-soaked cotton and pat gently to dry. Do not rub.
- Keep the area dry. Wear cotton panties and panty hose with a cotton crotch panel to allow moisture to evaporate.
- Eliminate certain foods from the diet—caffeinated drinks, chocolate, tomatoes, and beer. This may help.
- Most important, stop scratching. If necessary, apply a strong steroid ointment to the area to break the itch-scratch cycle.

LIVER DISORDERS

Located in the right upper abdomen, the liver is the body's largest solid organ, and one of the most complex. It has more than 500 separate functions, but its chief importance is as the center for the receipt and assimilation of food, including carbohydrates, proteins, fats, minerals, and vitamins. The liver also stores carbohydrates, regulates blood sugar levels, detoxifies drugs and substances harmful to the body, and produces important body chemicals, such as bile, blood proteins, urea, and clotting components. The liver lives up to its name—it is absolutely essential to human life.

Fortunately, the liver is protected from disease in several ways. It is capable of regeneration, meaning it can repair or replace injured tissue. Second, the liver is composed of large numbers of individual units that can take over for injured units indefinitely, or until the injury heals. However, the liver is subject to various inflammatory conditions that can injure and destroy individual cells and threaten the overall health of the organ.

Hepatitis

Hepatitis—inflammation of the liver—refers to the breakdown and dysfunction of the hepatocytes, the individual cells of the liver. One of the most common of liver diseases, hepatitis is caused primarily by viruses, although alcohol, drugs, and a variety of infections can also lead to liver inflammation. The most common hepatitis viruses are labeled A, B, and C. Other viruses, such as mononucleosis, can cause a mild hepatitis. Lupoid hepatitis is an autoimmune inflammation seen primarily in women.

Hepatitis can be acute and dramatic, or chronic and smoldering. It can clear up without a trace or leave severe scars that disrupt the functioning of the liver and block its blood flow, creating a serious condition called cirrhosis.

Viral Hepatitis—A, B, C, Delta, and E

Hepatitis A is acquired through ingesting food or water contaminated by sewage (the fecal-oral route). *Hepatitis B* is transmitted by infected blood or body fluids—the parenteral route—and is usually caused by contaminated blood products, sharing infected needles, or sexual intercourse with an infected person, particularly anal sex. *Hepatitis C* is spread primarily by the parenteral route but is less likely to be transmitted via intimate contact than hepatitis B. *Delta hepatitis* is caused by a highly specialized virus that affects liver cells only when hepatitis B is present; it increases the severity of the infection. *Hepatitis E* is acquired by the same route as hepatitis A. Rare in the United States, it is seen only in people from Asia, particularly India. It is notable for its extremely acute effects on pregnant women.

Symptoms

Viral hepatitis first shows up as a flulike illness characterized by extreme fatigue, fever, loss of appetite, and achiness. Urine may turn dark brown ("Coca-Cola" urine) and test positive for bile. This dark pigment is bilirubin, a breakdown product of the red blood cells, which are normally metabolized by the liver and excreted in the bile. When the kidneys and liver cannot remove the bilirubin, it remains in the blood and you develop jaundice, a yellow discoloration of the eyes and skin.

Diagnosis

A specific diagnosis of hepatitis is made by means of blood tests. These tests reflect the damage and destruction of the liver cells, and are the best way to monitor the progress of the disease. There are now individual tests to identify the specific type of hepatitis, although there are still a number of cases in which the cause cannot be definitely identified.

Treatment

There is no specific treatment for viral hepatitis. Rest, abstaining from alcohol, and adequate nutrition are all important in returning the liver to normal functioning. Hepatitis can vary from a mild, short-term illness to what is called fulminant hepatitis, a progressive destruction of the liver leading rapidly to coma and death. Most cases are somewhere between these two extremes, usually consisting of several weeks of symptoms, including jaundice, that reach a peak and then slowly return to normal. Some patients with hepatitis B or C never quite get over the infection and go on to develop chronic hepatitis. These people require special care and follow-up because of the danger of cirrhosis. In some cases, treatment with interferon, an antiviral substance, can enable the immune system to overcome the virus; it has worked in only about one-third of cases tested, however.

Hepatitis B carrier

In a person who is a carrier, the B virus resides in the liver cells without causing overt symptoms. The carrier is not ill, but he or she is capable of transmitting the virus to others. For example, the virus can be transmitted from a woman to her fetus in the uterus. Active and passive immunization of a baby born to a carrier mother can prevent a similar carrier state in the newborn.

Some adult carriers can develop immunity by interferon treatment.

Other Types of Hepatitis

Lupoid hepatitis

Lupoid hepatitis is a chronic hepatitis associated with autoimmune phenomena. The symptoms of the disease can be improved by treatment with corticosteroid medications.

Alcoholic hepatitis

This type of inflammation is caused by the toxic effects of alcohol. It can occur in its acute form, with symptoms of fever and jaundice, or it can be a chronic smoldering process that eventually leads to scarring and cirrhosis. Excessive alcohol consumption can also lead to fatty infiltration of the liver, which means fat is deposited in the liver cells. This condition can lead to liver swelling and discomfort in the right upper abdomen. Diabetes can also cause fatty infiltration.

Drug hepatitis

Certain medications can induce a hypersensitivity reaction in the liver. The drugs most commonly causing this condition are some blood pressure medications and medications controlling cholesterol, seizures, arthritis, and tuberculosis. Liver function tests done in the first few months after starting these drugs can identify the reaction, and alternative drugs can be substituted. Certain drugs kept past their expiration date, such as the antibiotic tetracycline, can degenerate into toxic compounds that damage the liver. Some drugs taken in large quantities are toxic to the liver—acetaminophen, for one.

How to Protect Your Liver

The most common serious infection of the liver is viral hepatitis. The most frequently contracted viruses are the "infectious" variety (known as hepatitis A), transmitted by the fecal-oral route, and the type of hepatitis transmitted through blood or blood products, hepatitis B or C, also known as serum hepatitis.

You can contract hepatitis A by drinking water contaminated by sewage. In the United States, the most common scenario is that campers or hikers drink water from a stream, thinking it is pure. Never drink from outdoor water sources, no matter how isolated the area. If necessary, purify the water before using. When traveling to countries where hepatitis A is common in the population, get a gamma globulin shot in advance of the trip. Gamma globulin can give you temporary immunity to hepatitis A and protect you for 3–6 months, depending on the dose. When you travel, ask your travel agent or the Department of Health whether this precaution is necessary.

Hepatitis B and C are generally more serious forms of the disease. Sensitive tests have all but eliminated hepatitis B and C from our blood supply, but posttransfusion hepatitis still occurs, caused by unidentified viruses. If you are having elective surgery, and might need a blood transfusion, ask your doctor about *autologous transfusion*. In this procedure, you donate the blood yourself, in advance of the operation.

Because some people are carriers of hepatitis B—the virus is in their bodies, even though they are not sick themselves—and because the hepatitis B virus is transmissible by intimate contact, including exchange of body fluids, always use barrier protection if you have sexual relations with anyone whose detailed medical and sexual history is unknown to you. And, obviously, never use a hypodermic needle that has been used by another person. There is now a very effective vaccine against hepatitis B. It is recommended for health care workers, patients receiving blood products (such as hemophiliacs), and spouses and intimate partners of hepatitis B carriers.

■ *Medications.* A number of commonly used drugs can cause liver damage in certain individuals. Whenever you are placed on a long-term prescription medication, particularly for high blood pressure, high cholesterol, seizures, or tuberculosis, ask your doctor about the possibility of toxicity to the liver and the need for periodic tests to check for liver damage. If these tests are recommended, make sure to have them done and that you are notified of the results. Most people who are going to have an adverse reaction to the medication will have it in the first few months after starting the drug.

■ *Toxins on the job.* Cleaning fluids, such as carbon tetrachloride, can induce severe liver damage if inhaled in sufficient amounts. Polyvinyl chloride, a substance produced in the manufacturing of plastics, also has been associated with liver damage. If you work in a cleaning establishment or a plastics factory, make sure that sufficient safeguards exist to prevent any chance of these toxins affecting your health.

Cirrhosis

Cirrhosis is a term used to indicate a condition in which the liver is progressively and irreversibly damaged by toxins or infection. In cirrhosis, normal liver tissue is replaced by scar tissue and areas of regenerating liver cells, leading to disruption of normal liver circulation. Blood does not flow freely through the liver, and the cells are poorly nourished. High pressure builds up in the portal system, the network of veins that carries blood from the intestines to the liver. This is called portal hypertension. Reversal of blood flow may cause the spleen to enlarge. Varices (enlarged veins) may develop in the esophagus and can rupture and bleed profusely. Other circulatory disruptions cause fluid and protein to accumulate in the peritoneal cavity, a condition called ascites.

Causes

The most common causes of cirrhosis are alcohol consumption and hepatitis. Rarer causes are described at the end of this section.

Most cases of cirrhosis appear after heavy, long-term alcohol ingestion or as the end stage of a case of hepatitis that has become chronic. Occasionally an individual with no remarkable prior history presents with cirrhosis, which is called cryptogenic cirrhosis.

Symptoms

Symptoms of cirrhosis are generally related to the inability of the liver to process bodily toxins and medications, and to manufacture proteins; to the pressure of ascites on abdominal organs; and to complications from high pressure in the portal blood system. Cirrhosis symptoms include loss of appetite, weight loss, fatigue, altered mental function (from agitation to coma), jaundice, bleeding disorders, fluid accumulation, severe gastrointestinal bleeding, and the development of tiny, spiderlike blood vessels under the skin.

Diagnosis

Physical examination reveals a small liver and an enlarged spleen. Ascites and jaundice may be present. Blood tests may reveal low levels of proteins and clotting factors. A liver-spleen scan shows the size of the liver and spleen. A liver biopsy—a piece of the liver removed and studied under a microscope—can give information about the cause of the cirrhosis because of typical cellular patterns. CT scan can be helpful in defining the anatomy and size of the liver, and enlargement of blood vessels.

Treatment

All toxins (like alcohol) and mind-altering medications must be discontinued. Cleansing and acidifying the colon with a compound called lactulose can remove nitrogenous compounds that contribute to hepatic coma. Bleeding esophageal varices can be thrombosed through endoscopic sclerotherapy. Portal hypertension can be reduced by operations that shunt the blood flow out of the portal network. These treatments can control some of the symptoms of cirrhosis, but there is no treatment to reverse the disease. The sad fact is that when the liver cell population falls below a critical mass, liver failure ensues and the patient will die. Some patients benefit from liver transplantation, but this procedure is limited by availability of organs and the complex medical care required to maintain a transplant.

Rare Conditions That Can Cause Cirrhosis

Primary biliary cirrhosis

Most commonly seen in middle-aged women, this is a rare condition in which the small bile ducts appear to be attacked and destroyed. The main symptom is severe itching, due to poor excretion of the bile acids. The cause appears to be an autoimmune phenomenon. Complications result from blockage of the bile flow and the development of scars on the liver, eventually leading to cirrhosis.

Hemochromatosis

This is an inherited (autosomal recessive) disease characterized by the accumulation of iron in the liver, pancreas, heart, skin, and other organs. The cause is the inability of the intestine to regulate the amount of iron absorbed from the diet. Premenopausal women are protected from its effects by menstrual blood loss, but postmenopausal women affected by the disease show high amounts of circulating and stored iron in the body. A liver biopsy will show the amount of iron and how much damage the liver has sustained. The condition can be controlled by removing blood from the body (phlebotomy) periodically to maintain the desired iron level.

Wilson's disease

This is a rare inherited disease caused by the accumulation of copper in the body, primarily in the brain and the liver. A young person who develops hepatitis without an obvious cause, like infection, should be checked for Wilson's disease. Symptoms may include tremors, seizures, and other neurological problems. Medications that bind and remove copper from the body can relieve symptoms; with proper treatment, the prognosis is good. Other family members, particularly siblings, should be tested for the disease.

Tumors of the Liver

Most tumors of the liver are malignant. Primary tumors, or hepatomas, arise from liver cells; secondary or metastatic tumors spread to the liver from another part of the body. In Africa and Asia, primary liver cell cancer is the leading cause of cancer death. In the United States it is an uncommon but extremely serious form of cancer that is one-third as likely to appear in women as in men.

Certain factors tend to predispose a person to primary liver cancer, including chronic viral hepatitis and damage from a toxin, usually alcohol.

Benign tumors of the liver rarely occur. The most common are hepatic adenomas, which are associated with long-term use of oral contraceptives, and hemangiomas. Hemangiomas are tumors composed of abnormal collections of blood vessels. These tumors usually produce no symptoms, and may be discovered when liver scans are done for other reasons. If they do produce symptoms—pain or internal bleeding—hemangiomas can be removed surgically. Otherwise, treatment is not needed.

Metastatic liver cancer is by far the most common form of liver cancer in the United States. It is easy to see why. The liver is like a gigantic sieve, filtering the blood coming from the digestive tract through the portal system and from the lung through the hepatic artery. Tumor cells from cancers of the stomach, breast, lung, pancreas, esophagus, gallbladder, and colon can all find their way to the liver, become lodged, and start to grow.

Symptoms
Malignant tumors of the liver may produce no symptoms until the disease is far advanced. The most common signs are pain in the right upper abdomen, loss of appetite and weight, general fatigue and weakness, nausea and vomiting, and jaundice.

Diagnosis
If liver cancer is suspected, the doctor will take blood tests. A CT scan can locate the tumor. A liver biopsy of the tumor site provides the definitive diagnosis. If it does not, laparoscopy, a small exploratory operation, a "mini lap," may be advised.

Treatment

Liver cancer is almost always fatal. In primary cancer of the liver cells, neither liver transplantation nor any chemotherapeutic regimen has been found to cure hepatoma. In rare cases when the tumor has been confined to a single site, successful surgical removal has been possible.

In metastatic liver cancer, the development of new tumors in the liver is a grave prognostic sign. Chemotherapy can shrink some tumors temporarily but will rarely destroy them completely. As with all chemotherapy decisions, the side effects of the treatment must be carefully weighed against the possible benefit.

THE LIVER BIOPSY

If you are being diagnosed for a liver ailment, your doctor may perform a liver biopsy, in which a small piece of liver tissue is removed and examined under a microscope. A biopsy permits direct examination of the cells and structures of the liver to differentiate types of hepatitis and tumors.

You will be given a local anesthetic and instructed to lie flat on your back. Your physician will insert a special biopsy needle between your ribs on the right side and remove a small sample of liver tissue for laboratory analysis. You will then be instructed to lie on your right side and be monitored for a certain amount of time, to eliminate any risk of hemorrhage.

A liver biopsy is quite safe and carries a minimum risk of side effects or bleeding.

GALLBLADDER AND BILE DUCT DISORDERS

A small, pear-shaped organ, the gallbladder stores bile, a complex substance produced by the liver. Bile contains bile acids (derived from cholesterol) and lecithin, chemicals required for the absorption of fat. It also contains cholesterol, bilirubin, and metabolized drugs and toxins that are being excreted from the body. The gallbladder removes water from the bile and concentrates it. When food containing fat is consumed, the gallbladder discharges the bile through the bile duct into the intestine.

The formation of gallstones (cholelithiasis) is the most common type of gallbladder disease.

Gallstones and Cholecystitis

Stones form in the gallbladder if the bile becomes concentrated enough to crystallize the cholesterol or the calcium bilirubinate found there. Gallstones are three times more common in women than in men, and the incidence increases with age. Not all gallstones consist of the same material. Cholesterol gallstones are the most common type; a small minority are made up of calcium salts. Often gallstones produce no symptoms. They may be detected when tests are done for abdominal symptoms, but the mere presence of the stones does not mean they are responsible for the symptoms. The most common problem caused by gallstones is cholecystitis, or inflammation of the gallbladder.

Cholecystitis commonly occurs when a stone gets stuck in the cystic duct, and the wall of the gallbladder becomes swollen and irritated. An attack of acute cholecystitis is usually precipitated by a meal containing fat, when the gallbladder, working hard, contracts vigorously and sends a stone into the cystic duct. (See Fig. 3.12)

Symptoms

If a stone lodges in the cystic duct, it produces painful contractions in the upper right area of the abdomen as the gallbladder tries to empty itself of the obstructing stone. Nausea and vomiting are common. If the stone begins to travel through the duct system, it produces severe pain, called biliary colic, which is felt in the right upper abdomen and sometimes around the ribs

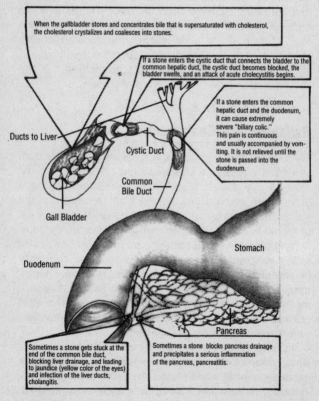

When the gallbladder stores and concentrates bile that is supersaturated with cholesterol, the cholesterol crystalizes and coalesces into stones.

If a stone enters the cystic duct that connects the bladder to the common hepatic duct, the cystic duct becomes blocked, the bladder swells, and an attack of acute cholecystitis begins.

If a stone enters the common hepatic duct and the duodenum, it can cause extremely severe "biliary colic." This pain is continuous and usually accompanied by vomiting. It is not relieved until the stone is passed into the duodenum.

Ducts to Liver

Cystic Duct

Common Bile Duct

Gall Bladder

Stomach

Duodenum

Pancreas

Sometimes a stone gets stuck at the end of the common bile duct, blocking liver drainage, and leading to jaundice (yellow color of the eyes) and infection of the liver ducts, cholangitis.

Sometimes a stone blocks pancreas drainage and precipitates a serious inflammation of the pancreas, pancreatitis.

Figure 3.12 Gallstones and Their Complications

to the right side of the back. This pain is comparable in severity to renal colic (kidney stones) and labor pains. If the stone passes through the ducts to the intestine, the pain is relieved dramatically. If the stone lodges at the end of the common bile duct, it can block the passage of bile from the liver, causing obstructive jaundice. It can also precipitate an infection in the bile duct system (cholangitis), or bring on an attack of acute pancreatitis. The possibility of these serious complications makes it imperative to remove the stone from the common bile duct (see treatment).

Chronic cholecystitis may develop in women who experience many episodes of gallbladder inflammation. The wall of the gallbladder thickens, affecting the cellular lining. The gallbladder no longer functions effectively, nor is it able to concentrate the bile.

Diagnosis
If your symptoms fit the clinical picture of cholecystitis, your physician will give you tests that are most helpful in confirming the diagnosis. These tests include an ultrasound of the abdomen, which can show stones in the gallbladder, and an HIDA scan, which reveals blockages in the flow of bile.

Treatment
The good news about gallstone disease is that it can be completely cured by removal of the gallbladder. This operation is called a *cholecystectomy*. A standard cholecystectomy is a major surgical procedure with a 6-to-8-week recovery time. It usually leaves a slanting scar in the right upper abdomen, under the rib cage.

In the late 1980's, a new procedure called *laparoscopic cholecystectomy* became available. This procedure uses multiple instruments introduced through several small incisions in the abdomen. The recovery time is much shorter than with the standard operation. Laparoscopic surgery is most useful for uncomplicated acute cases with little or no scarring around the gall-bladder. Since a laparoscopic procedure may have to be converted at any time during surgery to a standard operation, it should be done by a surgeon who has had extensive experience in standard cholecystectomies and specific training and experience in the laparoscopic technique.

If a stone becomes lodged in one of the ducts, it is extremely important to remove the obstructing object before severe complications ensue. In a standard cholecystectomy, the surgeon will explore the common bile duct to make sure that all the stones in the duct system are removed. If you have complications or you are too ill to withstand major surgery, you can be treated by sphincterotomy, a procedure using an instrument called an endoscope, which opens the muscles at the end of the common bile duct, releasing the stone.

Some cases of gallstone disease can be treated without surgery. Medication derived from bile acids can change the balance of chemicals in the bile and dissolve the crystallizing cholesterol. This treatment works best when there are many small stones and the gallbladder cells are functioning well in removing water from the bile. A good candidate for this treatment does not have severe symptoms or complications. It is also beneficial for those patients unwilling or unable to undergo surgery because of other medical problems. After the gallstones are dissolved, a maintenance dose of medication must be taken to keep the cholesterol from forming new stones.

Other Bile Duct Disorders

Sclerosing cholangitis is a rare disorder affecting the bile duct system. The walls of the duct become thickened and irregular, causing jaundice and infection. Sclerosing cholangitis sometimes is found in patients suffering from ulcerative colitis, one of the inflammatory bowel diseases.

Cancer of the biliary tract is very rare, but it can occur in the gallbladder, the large bile ducts, or the duct system in the liver. *Cancer of the gallbladder* occurs only in association with chronic gallbladder inflammation and may be found only when the gallbladder is removed in a cholecystectomy. As with many other intestinal cancers, these tumors do not cause symptoms, such as pain or jaundice, until they are well advanced, and cannot be removed successfully with surgery. At that point, treatment is usually palliative, directed at relieving symptoms.

DISORDERS OF THE PANCREAS

A large, complex gland located in the upper abdomen, behind the lower part of the stomach, the pancreas has two distinct functions. Scattered small groups of cells within the pancreas, called the islets of Langerhans, manufacture insulin and other essential hormones that regulate the body's sugar metabolism. Its second function is to produce enzymes required for the digestion of starch, fat, and protein. These enzymes are secreted in response to hormones signaled by the presence of food in the intestine. The enzymes flow into the duct system that joins the common bile duct as it empties into the duodenum. Because the drainage system of the liver is adjacent to the pancreas, conditions in the pancreas can affect the liver, causing jaundice and giving the first clue that something is wrong with the pancreas. Conversely, because the drainage ducts of the liver and the pancreas are connected, gallstones from the biliary ducts can interfere with pancreatic drainage and lead to pancreatic inflammation.

Acute Pancreatitis

Pancreatitis occurs when a chemical, toxin, pressure, or infection causes the enzyme-manufacturing cells of the pancreas to rupture, leading to irritation and swelling of the pancreatic tissue. The most common causes of acute pancreatitis are gallstone disease and excessive alcohol ingestion. Rarer instigators are the viral illness of mumps and high blood levels of certain fats, the triglycerides.

Symptoms
The main symptoms of acute pancreatitis are severe upper abdominal pain that often begins 12 to 24 hours after a large meal or a bout of heavy drinking, followed by vomiting, fever, and chills.

Diagnosis
The physical exam reveals severe tenderness in the upper abdomen. The diagnosis is confirmed by the finding of elevated levels of the enzymes amylase and lipase in the blood.

Treatment
The course of pancreatitis can range from mild pain to massive destruction of the pancreas and death. If you are suffering from acute pancreatitis, you will be hospitalized and all food intake will be stopped. The aim is to quiet the gland, stopping the flow of enzymes as much as possible. Food is given intravenously, and the stomach is drained with a tube to remove all stimuli to the pancreas. Severe cases will require complex care in the

intensive care unit. The most important element of long-term treatment is to eliminate the cause of the pancreatitis by removing the gallstones, or stopping alcohol ingestion, or controlling blood lipids.

Cancer of the Pancreas

Pancreatic cancer is one of the more common cancers, ranking just behind cancers of the lung, colon, and breast. It is perhaps more frequent in people who smoke, drink heavily, or have chronic pancreatitis or diabetes, but it can and does occur in individuals with none of those factors. It is less common in women than in men.

Symptoms

The signs of pancreatic cancer depend on the location of the tumor. Most of these cancers produce no symptoms until the cancer has spread outside the gland. One exception is when the tumor is located near the common bile duct or the main pancreatic duct. When the liver ducts are blocked, the liver malfunctions and jaundice can develop; when the pancreatic duct is blocked, malabsorption with diarrhea can occur. In most cases, however, the common symptoms of lack of appetite, weight loss, nausea and vomiting, and abdominal pain occur after the cancer has spread elsewhere in the body.

Diagnosis

A physical exam may reveal an upper abdominal mass. Liver tests may show signs of bile duct obstruction. A course of pancreatic enzyme medication may stop the diarrhea, pointing to the pancreas as the cause.

Ultrasound or a CT scan can locate the tumor and determine whether the duct systems are dilated, and if there are enlarged nodes or metastatic tumors in the liver.

Treatment

The survival rate for those with pancreatic cancer is poor. In rare cases, surgery on the pancreas is successful in removing the tumor. More commonly, because the tumor is far advanced, treatment consists of reestablishing the flow of bile and pancreatic secretion into the intestine by placing drains through the tumor via an endoscope or by a surgical bypass operation. There is no chemotherapeutic regimen developed to date that eradicates pancreatic cancer.

EDITORS AND CONTRIBUTORS

MEDICAL CO-EDITORS

ROSELYN PAYNE EPPS, M.D., M.P.H., M.A., F.A.A.P., is an expert at the National Institutes of Health, Bethesda, Maryland, and a Professor at Howard University College of Medicine, Washington, D.C. She is recognized nationally and internationally in areas of health policy and research, health promotion and disease prevention, and medical education and health service delivery. As a pioneer and leader in numerous professional and community organizations, she served, in 1991, as the first African-American president of AMWA and the founding president of the AMWA Foundation.

SUSAN COBB STEWART, M.D., F.A.C.P., is an internist and gastroenterologist, and is presently Associate Medical Director at J. P. Morgan in New York, where she delivers general medical care, specialty consultations, and preventive services. She is Clinical Assistant Professor of Medicine at SUNY, Brooklyn. Since serving as President of AMWA in 1990, Dr. Stewart has continued to help AMWA shape and focus its mission in the area of women's health.

CONTRIBUTORS

Tamara G. Bavendam, M.D., F.A.C.S., is Director of Female Urology at the University of Washington School of Medicine in Seattle, where she is an Assistant Professor of Urology. She has developed a multispecialty, multidisciplinary approach to urological problems in women.

Jean L. Fourcroy, M.D., Ph.D., is a urologist with a primary interest in male reproductive endocrinology and toxicology. She is medical officer in the Division of Endocrinology and Metabolic Drug Products of the Food and Drug Administration. She is also an Assistant Professor of Surgery at the University of Health Sciences—F. Edward Hebert

School of Medicine and the founder of Women in Urology. Dr. Fourcroy served as AMWA President in 1996.

Sandra P. Levison, M.D., F.A.C.P., is a Professor and Associate Chair of the Department of Medicine, Chief of the Division of Nephrology of the Medical College of Pennsylvania and Hahnemann University, and serves as Program Director of the Nephrology Fellowship Program and Co-Director of the Dialysis Unit. She is a founding member and past president of Women in Nephrology.

Katherine A. O'Hanlan, M.D., F.A.C.O.G., F.A.C.S., is an Assistant Professor of Gynecology and Obstetrics at Stanford University School of Medicine in California and Associate Director of the Gynecological Cancer Service at Stanford Medical Center.

INDEX

Abdominal aorta, 72
Abortion, 33–35, 61
ACE inhibitors, 96–97, 110, 115
Acetaminophen, 191
Achalasia, 142, 151, 152
Acute appendicitis, 168–170
Acute kidney failure, 95–97
Acute pancreatitis, 204–205
Adenomatous polyps, 178
AIDS, 11, 26, 102, 104, 113
Alcohol, 52, 138–139, 158, 160
Alcoholic hepatitis, 191
Amebiasis, 164
Amenorrhea, 52–53
Anal fissure, 182–183
Anal itching, 185, 187
Anorectal disorders, 181–183
Anorexia nervosa, 131
Anoscopy, 155

Antibiotics, 16, 17, 55, 59, 80–83, 115
Anus, 128
Appendicitis, 168–170
Aspirin, 158
Atrophic gastritis, 156–158
Autologous transfusion, 192
Autosomal dominant polycystic kidney disease (ADPKD), 105–107

Bacterial gastroenteritis, 164
Bacterial vaginosis, 59
Barium enema, 154
Barium X-ray, 150, 154
Barrett's esophagus, 144, 146
Bartholin's glands, 3
Bethesda system, 14, 36
Biliary colic, 200
Biliary tract cancer, 203
Birth control, 13, 19–33
Bladder, 70–73
Bladder cancer, 75
Bladder infection, 80–81

Bladder training, 92, 94
Bladder tumors, 108–109
Bleeding, excessive, 54
Bloody urine, 77–78
Bone density test, 52
Breast cancer, 23, 51
Bromocriptine, 57
Bulimia, 131

CA-125 blood test, 42, 43
Caffeine, 158, 160
Calcium, 50, 52, 74, 85
Calcium channel blockers, 84
Cardiovascular disease, 23, 50, 51
Cecum, 128, 168
Celiac (nontropical) sprue, 167–168
Cervical cancer, 14, 27, 36–39
Cervical cap, 21, 25–27
Cervical conization, 39
Cervix, 3, 6
Chlamydia, 11, 16, 55
Cholecystectomy, 201, 202
Cholecystitis, 199–201
Cholecystokinin, 129
Cholesterol, 23, 51
Chronic kidney failure, 95–97
Chronic pancreatitis, 168
Chyme, 129

Cirrhosis, 189, 193–196
Clitoris, 2, 3, 5
Colon, 128, 129, 140, 154, 168, 169
Colonoscopy, 155, 169
Colorectal cancer, 179–181
Colorectal surgeons, 141
Colposcopy, 60–61
Computerized axial tomography (CT) scan, 121
Condoms, 11, 13, 21, 22, 26–29
Constipation, 92, 94, 134–135, 173, 177, 183
Continuous ambulatory peritoneal dialysis (CAPD), 98, 100–101
Contraception (see Birth control)
Corpus luteum, 11
Cramps, 53–54
Crohn's disease, 170–173
Cryotherapy, 60
Cysteine, 86
Cystitis, 80–82
Cystometry, 122–123
Cystoscopy, 84, 122

Defecation, 129–130
Diabetes mellitus, 23, 96, 109–110, 117, 191
Dialysis, 98–100

Diaphragm, 21, 25, 26, 93
Diarrhea, 53, 54, 134, 164–165
Diet, 136–140
Diethylstilbestrol (DES), 43
Dilation and curettage (D&C), 41, 54, 61, 62
Dimethyl sulfoxide, 84
Diverticular disease, 175–178
Drug hepatitis, 191
Duodenum, 126, 129, 163
Dysentery, 163
Dyspepsia, 132–133
Dysphagia, 143, 145, 150

Eclampsia, 116, 117
Ectopic pregnancy, 22, 44–46
Elective abortion, 33
Electrolytes, 70, 72, 119
Electrosurgery, 39
Emotional changes, 50, 54
Endocrine system, 12
Endometrial biopsy, 52
Endometrial cancer, 22, 23, 39–41, 51
Endometrial hyperplasia, 40
Endometriosis, 46–48, 52, 62
Endometrium, 3, 7, 11, 22

Endoscopic retrograde cholangiopancreatography (ERCP), 155
Endoscopy, 146, 150, 159
End-stage renal disease (ESRD), 97, 110
Enuresis (bedwetting), 90
Erosive gastritis, 157
Esophageal cancer, 142, 144, 149–150
Esophageal disorders, 142–156
Esophagogastroduodenoscopy (EGD), 155
Esophagus, 126
Estrogen, 2–3, 7, 8, 11, 12, 20, 22, 40–41, 50–52, 85, 90, 91, 94, 95
Exercise, 138

Fallopian tubes, 6, 8, 9, 32, 44–46
Family physicians, 18
Fasting cholesterol test, 52
Fecal incontinence, 186
Feces, 129
Fertilization, 7, 9, 11
Fetal genitalia, 4
Fiber, 139–140, 175
Fibroids, 48–49, 52, 62
Fistula, 182
Focal glomerulosclerosis (FGS), 102, 103, 113

Follicle-stimulating hormone (FSH), 11
Freezing techniques, 39, 60

Gallbladder, 128
Gallbladder and bile duct disorders, 199–203
Gallbladder cancer, 203
Gallstones, 199–202
Gastritis, 156–158
Gastrocolic reflex, 130
Gastroenteritis, 156, 163–164
Gastroesophageal reflux disease (GERD), 143–149
Gastrointestinal pain, 130, 132
Gastroplasty, 171
Giardiasis, 164
GI series, 154–156, 159
Glans, 4
Glomerulonephritis, 77, 102, 111
Glomerulus, 71
Gluten, 167–168
Gonads (sex glands), 12
Gonorrhea, 11, 16, 55

Health care practitioners, 17–18
Heartburn, 132–133, 145, 146
Helicobacter pylori, 157, 159–160
Hemangiomas, 197

Hematuria, 77–78
Hemochromatosis, 196
Hemodialysis, 980
Hemorrhoids, 183–185
Heparin, 84
Hepatic adenomas, 197
Hepatitis, 188–193
Hepatologists, 141
Herpes, 11, 16
Hiatal hernia, 146
Hiccups, 154
High blood pressure, 23, 74, 95, 110–111, 115–117
Hormone replacement therapy, 40, 46, 50–52, 94
Hot flashes, 49–50
Human immunodeficiency virus (HIV), 58, 103, 104, 113
Human papillomavirus (HPV), 11, 16–17, 36, 43
Hydrochloric acid, 129
Hydronephrosis, 114
Hyperplastic polyps, 178
Hypothalamus, 11, 12
Hysterectomy, 39, 41, 46, 48, 49, 61–66
Hysteroscopy, 65–66

Ibuprofen, 75
Ileonal anastomosis, 172
Ileostomy, 172
Ileum, 126, 129, 154, 163

Imaging techniques,
    120–123
Immunosuppression, 102
Implants, contraceptive,
    21, 23–24
Incontinence, 72, 89–95
Indigestion, 132–133,
    161
Infections, urinary
    system, 79–82, 115
Infertility, 16, 46, 48
Inflammatory bowel
    disease (IBD),
    170–173
Inherited kidney disease,
    105–107
Injections, contracep-
    tive, 21, 25
Internists, 17
Interstitial cystitis, 78,
    83–85
Intestinal disorders,
    163–187
Intrauterine devices
    (IUDs), 21, 22, 30–31
Intravenous
    pyelography, 120–121
Irritable bladder, 74,
    82–83
Irritable bowel
    syndrome, 173–175
Irritations and
    inflammations, urinary
    system, 82–85

Jejunum, 126, 129, 154,
    163

Kidney biopsy, 120
Kidney disease,
    105–107, 117
Kidney failure (renal
    failure), 95–100
Kidney infection, 81–82
Kidneys, 70, 73
Kidney transplantation,
    103–105
Kidney tumors, 108

Labia majora and
    minora, 3
Labioscrotal swelling, 4
Lactose intolerance, 167
Laparoscopy, 33, 46,
    47, 63, 66–67,
    201–202
Large intestine, 128,
    129, 163
Laser therapy, 39, 67
Laxatives, 177
Levonorgestrel, 23
Lithotripsy, 88
Liver, 128
Liver cancer, 51, 196–
    198
Liver disorders, 23,
    188–198
Loop electrosurgical
    excision procedure
    (LEEP), 67–68
Lupoid hepatitis, 188,
    191
Lupus, 111–112, 117
Luteinizing hormone
    (LH), 11

Magnetic resonance imaging (MRI), 121–122
Malabsorption disorders, 166–168, 171
Menopause, 3, 8, 49–52
Menstrual cycle, 8, 11
Menstrual problems, 52–54
Menstruation, 2–3, 7
Mifepristone, 35
Minimal change disease, 102
Miscarriage, 33
Mononucleosis, 188
Motility disorders, 142, 151–153
Myomectomy, 48, 49

Naproxen, 75
Nausea, 130–131
Nephrologists, 76
Nephron, 70–71
Nephrotic syndrome, 100, 102–103, 112, 113
Noncancerous breast disease, 22
Nonsteroidal anti-inflammatory drugs (NSAIDs), 54, 57, 74–75, 158
Nurse-midwives, 18
Nurse practitioners,18

Obesity, 137, 171
Obstetrician-gynecologists, 17

Oophorectomy, 41
Oral contraceptives, 20–23, 57, 85
Organ transplantation, 103–105, 110
Osteoporosis, 50, 51
Ovarian cancer, 22, 41–42
Ovarian cysts, 22, 24, 42–43
Ovaries, 6, 7
Ovulation, 7, 8, 11
Oxalate, 74, 85

Pancreas, 128
disorders of, 203–206
transplantation, 110
Papanicolaou, George, 14
Pap test, 13–16, 36–39, 52
Parasitic infections, 164
Pelvic examination, 13, 14, 52
Pelvic inflammatory disease (PID), 31, 55
Penis, 2, 5
Pepsin, 129, 158
Peptic stricture, 142, 144
Peptic ulcer, 158–160
Peptides, 12
Perianal abscess, 181
Periodic abstinence, 21, 22, 31–32
Peritoneal dialysis, 98, 100–101
Peritonitis, 168

Phenazopyridine hydrochloride, 83, 84
Pituitary gland, 11, 12
Polycystic kidney disease, 95–96, 105–107
Polyps, colon, 178–179
Post-streptoccal glomerulonephritis, 102
Potassium, 70, 71, 96
Preeclampsia, 116, 117
Pregnancy, 113–117, 149
Premenstrual syndrome (PMS), 55–57
Primary amenorrhea, 52, 53
Primary biliary cirrhosis, 195
Proctologists, 141
Proctoscopy, 155, 180
Progesterone, 7, 11, 12, 20, 30, 31
Progestin, 20, 23, 24, 50–51
Prostaglandin inhibitors, 54
Prostaglandins, 53–54
Prostate gland, 12
Puberty, 2, 3
Pyelonephritis, 81

Radical partial vulvectomy, 44
Rape, 57–58
Rectum, 75, 77, 79, 128
Reflux esophagitis, 131, 143–149

Regurgitation, 131, 151
Renal artery, 72
Renal artery stenosis, 110–111
Renal colic, 78, 201
Rhythm method, 31–32
RU-486, 35
Rumination, 131

Scleroderma, 142, 151–152
Sclerosing cholangitis, 202–203
Secondary amenorrhea, 52, 53
Secretin, 129
Semen, 3
Sexually transmitted diseases (STDs), 10–11, 13, 16–17, 25, 26, 55, 58, 112–113
Sickle cell disease, 111
Small intestine, 126
Smoking, 23, 50, 52, 75, 94, 139
Sodium, 70, 71, 96
Spastic disorders, 142, 152–153
Speculum, 14, 60
Sperm, 3
Spermicides, 21, 22, 27, 29
Sponge, contraceptive, 21, 22, 29–30
Spontaneous abortion, 33
Spontaneous incontinence, 90

Sterilization, 21, 22, 32–33
Steroids, 84, 102
Stomach, 126, 129
Stomach disorders, 156–162
Stones, 78, 85–88
Stress incontinence, 89
Syphilis, 11, 17, 112
Systemic disorders, 109–113

Testosterone, 3, 12
Therapeutic abortion, 33–34
Thromboembolism (blood clots), 23
Traveler's diarrhea, 165–166
Trichomonas, 17
Trigonitis, 82
Tubal ligation, 21, 22, 32
Tubule, 71

Ulcerative colitis, 170–173
Ultrasound, 42, 43, 48, 68, 120, 121
Upper gastrointestinal series (UGIS), 146
Uremia, 97, 113
Ureters, 70–72
Urethra, 3, 70, 71, 72, 75, 77, 79
Urethral syndrome, 82
Urethritis, 16, 82
Urge incontinence, 89

Uric acid, 85, 86
Urinalysis, 118–119
Urinary incontinence, 72, 89–95
Urinary urgency and frequency, 76, 78, 80
Urination, 71
Urine culture, 119
Urodynamics, 122–123
Urogenital membrane, 4
Urologists, 76
Uterine fibroids, 22, 48–49
Uterus, 3, 6, 7

Vacuum curettage, 34
Vagina, 3, 6
cancer of, 43
dryness, 50, 52
Vaginal cones, 93
Vaginitis, 58–59
Vagus nerve, 154
Vasectomy, 21
Vena cava, 72
Viral gastroenteritis, 163–164
Viral hepatitis, 189–193
Vomiting, 130–132, 164
Vulva, 3
Vulvar cancer, 13, 43–44

Water consumption, 72–73, 81, 83, 88, 92
Wilson's disease, 196
Withdrawal method, 21

Yeast infection, 59–60